TABLE OF CONTENTS

Dear reader,

Welcome to our third edition of Martial Arts Magazine Australia. We value your unwavering support as we worked towards putting this issue together.

Writers from across Australia have submitted articles showcasing their style, their training, and their dedication. I hope that you will enjoy this issue's content as much as the team here at MAMA have.

As we move into 2024 and the year of the dragon, we look towards the symbolism that is shared and is common across many different styles of Martial Arts as well as the significance of the Year of the Dragon and what that means to us. If your own style has a symbol we have neglected to include please let us know. We want to learn about you and your practice and share the knowledge throughout our community.

With Christmas gone and the new year ahead - what are your new year resolutions? Would you like to attend more classes, learn another style, compete in a tournament, advance to the next rank or become more proficient in what you can already do?

People come to study martial arts for many different reasons, and just as varied are the reasons they keep practicing. What are yours and has your motivation changed from the day you began?

Everyone's journey is unique and no two people will ever be on the exact same path. We are always keen to hear and share your stories, you never know who your words will inspire to do better.

Until next time, happy reading!

Yours sincerely
Vanessa McKay

CAN YOU IMAGINE WHAT I WOULD DO IF I COULD DO ALL I CAN?

~SUN TZU~

2024
YEAR OF THE
DRAGON

Harness the Mighty Dragon

Making the Most of 2024

by Gary Chen

Every twelve years, the Chinese zodiac reaches its peak intensity with the powerful, celebrated Year of the Dragon. 2024 marks the next lunar cycle welcoming back the noble dragon. Unlike any other zodiac animal, the dragon is a mythical composite creature encompassing multiple auspicious beasts – commanding respect across Eastern cultures as the ultimate symbol of strength, fortune and divine blessing.

The upcoming dragon year holds substantial meaning for people worldwide. Those born under dragon signs identify deeply with the dragon's attributes. People of all backgrounds participate in festivities honouring the dragon's qualities. The dragon's blessed energy makes 2024 an opportune time to pursue ambitious goals or establish new enterprises. Regardless of one's zodiac animal, anyone can adopt the dragon's venerable virtues to channel transformative energy into daily life. By understanding the dragon's cultural symbolism, embracing dragon-themed celebrations, and exemplifying dragon energy, people worldwide can maximise fortune in 2024 and beyond.

The Dragon in Eastern Symbolism

In China, the long or imperial dragon is distinguished from lesser dragons by its five claws.

This celestial beast controls rainfall and storms, representing the yang masculine force complementing the yin feminine. As a divine bringer of water, the Chinese dragon balances fire and water. Its sinuous form reflects supple strength through soft power – using flow instead of force.

In Feng Shui systems, the East cardinal direction governs family and health. Associated with sunrise, spring and rebirth, this highly auspicious direction belongs to the ascending dragon. The paired dragon and phoenix represent an ideal balance between yin and yang energetics. Images of these dual creatures denote harmony between apparent opposites – light and dark, fire and water. Energetically, dragon and phoenix symbols help to integrate disparate aspects of the self or environment through synergistic unity.

Dragon symbolism also includes wisdom, longevity and ethereality, transcending the mundane world. Chinese dragons confer blessings during celebratory occasions. Various numbers of imperial dragons appear on robes indicating royal status. From ancient artifacts to contemporary performances, dragons permeate Chinese culture as the epitome of fortune and strength.

The Dragon's Personality

Those born in dragon years are said to share common traits like the dragon's fiery confidence and zeal. As magical creatures standing apart from other earthly animals, dragon year babies are touted as exceptional from birth. Their family may consider them destined for greatness before accomplishing anything! But high expectations spur these entitled dynamos towards actual success.

As fearless dreamers unencumbered by self-limiting beliefs, Year Dragons often achieve highly creative, entrepreneurial breakthroughs. But they shun mundane work, lacking opportunities for bold self-expression or leadership. Tigers and Monkeys especially annoy the showy Dragon by stealing their spotlight! Less impetuous Oxes and Roosters help balance the Dragon's grandiose, impatient nature through practical planning. In relationships, supportive partners must juggle encouraging the Dragon's lofty ambitions with keeping them grounded.

Above all, those born under Dragon signs exude charisma and bravado. Remember dragons are regional guardians safeguarding the innocent and destroying wickedness with righteous power. Dragons embrace this archetype. They often display greater idealism compared to other more cynical signs, believing themselves to be on a heroic life quest.

Overall, the dragon birth year marks babies for vibrant, visionary destinies full of daring adventures leading to fame and fortune.

Celebrating The Dragon Year

The Dragon Year excites widespread festivity, celebrating this preeminent zodiac sign. Events feature dragon theming, costumes and mascots highlighting the dragon's qualities everyone hopes to capture. People don capes, headdresses and face paint, resembling the dragon's whiskers and claws. Dragon dancing, parades and processions draw crowds who touch colourful models for good luck. Homes and businesses display dragon imagery to infuse spaces with the dragon's vibrant energy. Parents even drape babies in dragon swaddling clothes for health, success and protection.

These public celebrations tap into beloved mythology with deep, layered meaning. Legend holds the divine dragon Shenlong grants wishes and dispenses fortune. Festivities invite Shenlong's blessings into communities as an honoured guest. Dragon imagery wards off malicious spirits, clears stagnant energy, and ushers in renewal. People reflect on the past dragon year's events and set optimistic goals for the twelve years ahead during this reflective transition cycle.

Year Dragons hold lavish birthday parties capped with wishes made under dragon symbols.

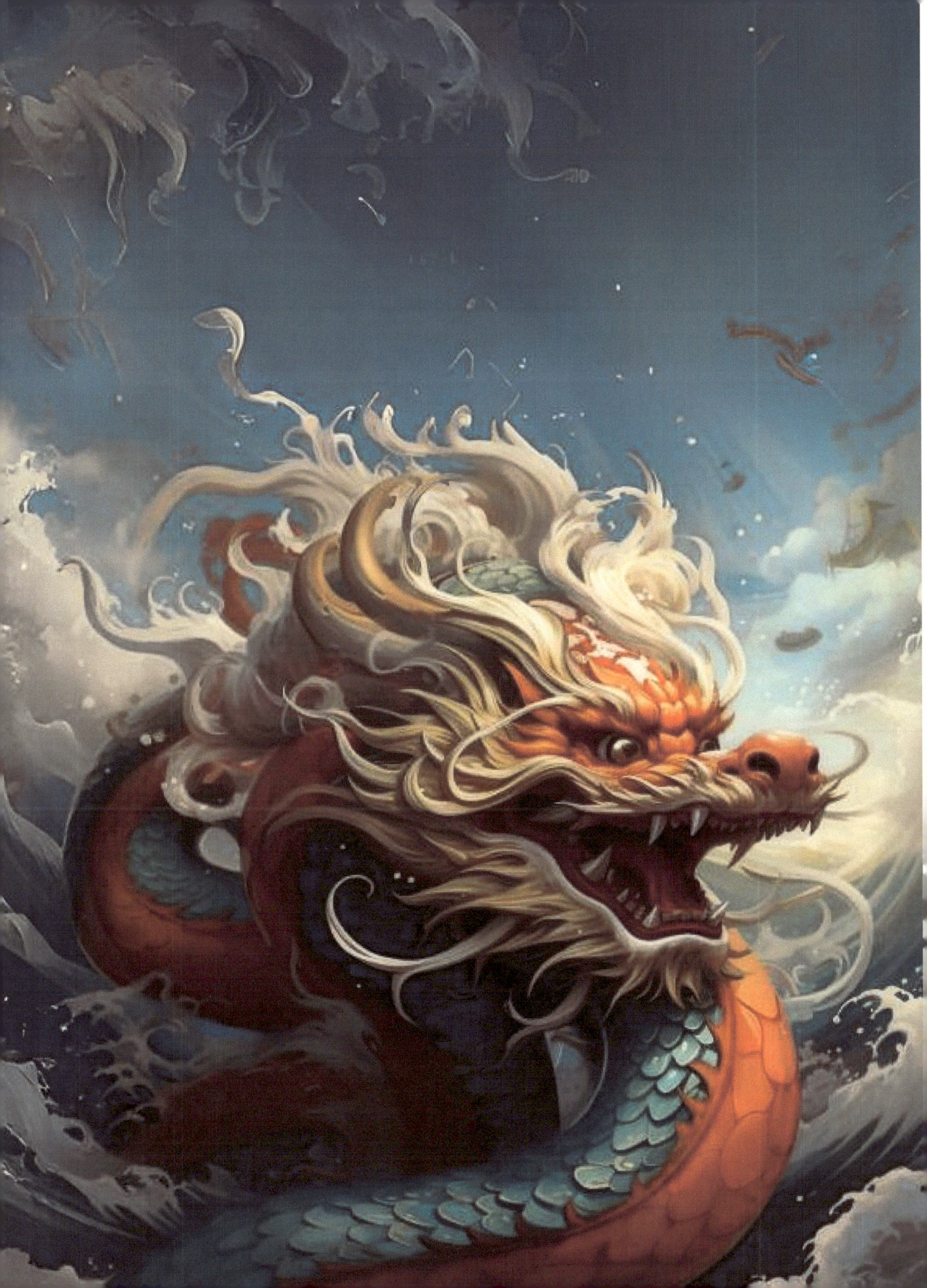

They don dragon regalia and claim gifts, in multiples of lucky number eight. Red dragon decor symbolises flaming ambition, wealth, and prestige. These new year celebrations recognise the individual's entry into a destined phase under the dragon's glorious guardianship. Young Year Dragons prepare to spread their wings.

A Fortuitous Year

Beyond celebrating those born under the sign, Dragon Years bless all new pursuits and relationships through association with dragon might. The powerful dragon energy makes it an extremely fortuitous time to launch major life initiatives or establish new commitments. Examples include:

Business Ventures
- Founding startups and small businesses
- Forming partnerships and corporations
- Investing in commercial real estate or properties
- Pursuing new ideas and creative projects

Life Milestones
- Engagement and marriage commitments for lasting union
- Conceiving children who will inherit the dragon's luck
- Moving into new homes associated with prosperity

Education Goals
- Enrollment into new schools and academic programs
- Taking licensing examinations and board exams
- Earning sought-after degrees, certifications and qualifications.

The Dragon Year's momentum propels new endeavours to amplified success compared to other timeframes lacking the dragon's fiery leadership essence. This aligns human activities to ascendant wood energy governed by the vernal East cardinal direction. Just as spring brings renewed possibilities for growth after winter's stagnation, the Dragon Year saves stalled projects and relationships. People capitalise on this surge by launching stalled initiatives now primed to manifest new potentials.

Overall, the dragon's auspicious influence lowers barriers and resistance towards actualising ambitious life plans. Things naturally fall into place this year through creative synergies and serendipitous timing. People worldwide ride 2024s intensified dragon wave as fortuitous timing for major decisions. They actualise this pulse wise cycle's optimum window for conceiving big ideas assured to prosper under the dragon's glowing patronage.

Channelling the Dragon

Daily Integration
Beyond simply celebrating the Lunar New Year, channelling dragon energy helps actualise personal goals. People worldwide can integrate dragon attributes as lasting life philosophies for success, independent of their animal sign. Some ideals to embrace include:

Noble Confidence

The dragon exemplifies self-assuredness without arrogance. This ESTJ* personality type stays grounded through high ethical standards, not egoism. Year Dragons feel comfortable taking authority yet wield power judiciously. Emulate their secure self-reliance, resisting overconfidence.

Might with Wisdom

Legendary dragons like Shenlong make enlightened decisions, destroying only wickedness with moral discernment. Before acting, consider long-term consequences like the farsighted dragon. Combine courage with wisdom.

Flexibility

The dragon's serpentine physicality represents transforming force: power with suppleness. Water governs the dragon's liquid strength. In confronting challenges, adjust approaches fluidly without compromising core integrity. Flow around obstacles as water carves stone.

Creativity over Convention

Eastern dragons transcend traditional animal forms as magical composites. Their multi-natured gifts break rigid paradigms through integrating apparent opposites. Take inspiration to go beyond either/or thinking through inclusive solutions.

Visionary Guidance

The divine dragon's higher vantage point allows for a clear-sighted perspective that is unavailable at ground level.

When facing decisions, take the dragon's elevated viewpoint. Envision long-range consequences before acting. Consult mentors for aerial guidance.

By integrating such ideals learned from the dragon's symbolic legacy, anyone can achieve amplified success consistent with the noble dragon's towering standards. Its blessing lifts endeavours above past limitations into awakened potential. Allow the lunar new year's intensified dragon energy to penetrate awareness fully, so this sign's majestic strengths animate all activity year-round. Then harness each year's possibilities, knowing the ascendant dragon perpetually oversees from awakened dominions, ready to gift those demonstrating virtue and wisdom.

*The Supervisor (Extroverted, Sensing, Thinking, Judging) **Chinese New Year falls on February 10th, 2024.*

Dragons: 2024, 2012, 2000,1988,1976, 1964

Rabbit: 2023, 2011, 1999, 1987, 1975, 1963

Tiger: 2022, 2010, 1998, 1986, 1974, 1962

Ox: 2021, 2009, 1997, 1985, 1973, 1961

Rat: 2020, 2008, 1996, 1984, 1972, 1960

Pig: 2019, 2007, 1995, 1983, 1971, 1959

Dog: 2018, 2006, 1994, 1982, 1970, 1958

Rooster: 2017, 2005, 1993, 1981,1969, 1957

Monkey:2016, 2004, 1992, 1980, 1968, 1956

Ram: 2027, 2015, 2003, 1991, 1979, 1967

Horse: 2026, 2014, 2002, 1990, 1978, 1966

Beyond Binary: The Octagon of Martial Arts Movement and Training
by Benjamin Ward

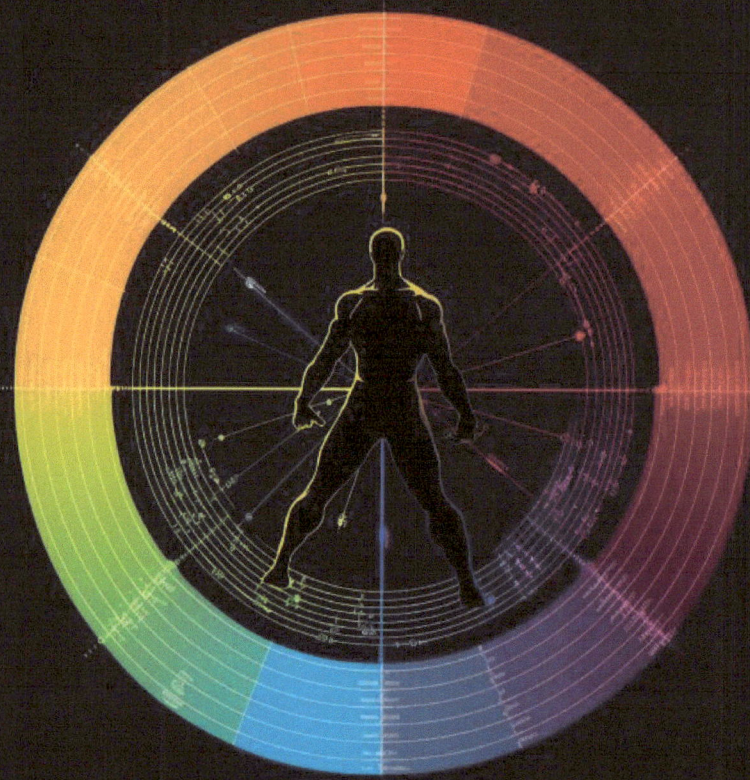

In martial arts, the concept of movement extends beyond simple distinctions like diagonal left, diagonal right, backward diagonal left, and backward diagonal right. When engaging in forward offensive or retreating defensive drills, individuals typically stand in a frontal position and signal left or right to strategically move either up the hall for offensive maneuvers or down the hall defensively during retreat. This approach introduces a fresh and effective drill for training.

To enhance individual combat practice, it is beneficial to move beyond the limited binary of two directions (forward or backward). A more comprehensive approach involves creating a drill that appears virtually indistinguishable to observers across a hall. This drill incorporates signaling movements in all four diagonal directions, allowing the student to respond both offensively and defensively, thereby increasing the complexity and effectiveness of the practice.

However when working with a towel in the wind on the clothesline, there was forward and backward as well. No doubt there would be left and right gaining no offensive or defensive ground.

The limitation to eight directions in martial arts is grounded in practicality. Attempting to execute precise movements, such as adjusting a stance by a single degree, like 270, 269, or 253 degrees, becomes impractical due to the inherent limitations of gross motor movements in the human body through space. Unlike the dexterity of fingers or the simplicity of a line on paper, such nuanced adjustments are challenging to implement effectively in physical practice.

Another reason for the limitation to eight directions is the practical need to focus on specific aspects rather than attempting to study everything simultaneously. Instead of a binary approach with just two directions, the more complex task of signing in four directions becomes quadratic in nature. To categorize these eight directions, we can refer to them as spectrums, drawing an analogy from spectrum analysis in science. This term implies examining a small frame of information to derive more comprehensive conclusions.

Anticipating an opponent's actions in a sparring situation, without the need for reactive responses, is comparable to moving in a perpetually straight line—a horizon that remains consistently distant and predictable, following a predetermined path. Conceptually, envisioning this predictability within the context of the eight directions forms an octagon shape, where a discernible horizon is positioned ahead of each of these predetermined paths. Despite our inclination to simplify, engaging in a sparring match is akin to facing a dynamic and unpredictable force, often likened to a random number generator by mathematicians due to the complexity of the human mind.

Engaging in patterns of movement involves not only straightforward and backward steps but also diagonal shifts in various directions, adding complexity. When incorporating lateral movements, such as circling to the left around an opponent, the potential combinations of movement and direction become virtually limitless. This diversity in motion creates an ever-changing and dynamic scenario every time one engages with an opponent.

The Zen philosophy, embodying the freedom aspect in Japanese, diverges from the symbolic representation of close-quarter combat and real-life fighting situations. It doesn't conform to the conventional eight directions confined within the conceptual boundaries of an octagon.

Engaging in martial arts training involves a degree of simplification. While diverse workouts contribute to overall preparation for a grading, some repetitive tasks or workloads become necessary, especially when training for a demanding grading like a second dan. Personally, during my journey to achieve my second dan, I faced the challenge of balancing work responsibilities and bills, which significantly reduced the time I could allocate to training. Shifting from a previous schedule of eight hours a day, six days a week, except for a paper run, forced me to make my training more efficient within the constraints of limited time and reduced planning availability.

As a result, there was a need for simplification, particularly in meeting the requirements for a second dan. This involved intensifying workouts, focusing on prioritized training in classes, incorporating active recovery work, emphasizing strength and cardio training, and dedicating time to preliminaries, sparring, and grade kata. These streamlined components became the essential focus of the training regimen for the second dan grading.

Simplifying the fundamental principles of movement in real-life combat and sparring can be likened to the preparation for a grading. It involves narrowing one's focus within martial arts and diligently pursuing specific goals, much like going to the gym three times a week to consistently follow the same workout routine and observe strength gains over time. The decision to simplify training is driven by constraints on time and increased responsibilities in other aspects of life, coupled with the need to concentrate on meeting grading requirements.

I began training in Zen Do Kai freestyle karate at age 13 and achieved my shodan-ho in 2001. I then studied two years of Wing Chun Kung fu while attending University. Upon returning to the Sunshine Coast I commenced training in Anderson Bushi Kai and achieved my rank of Nidan in 2013. I am currently sitting on the rank of Nidan with the title of Dai Sempai and continue to train in Anderson Bushi Kai at Coolum beach on the Sunshine Coast. I am 38 years old. Club: Anderson bushi kai -Sei Do Kai dojo - Coolum Beach, Sunshine Coast, QLD Club Contact: https://abksunshinecoast.com/

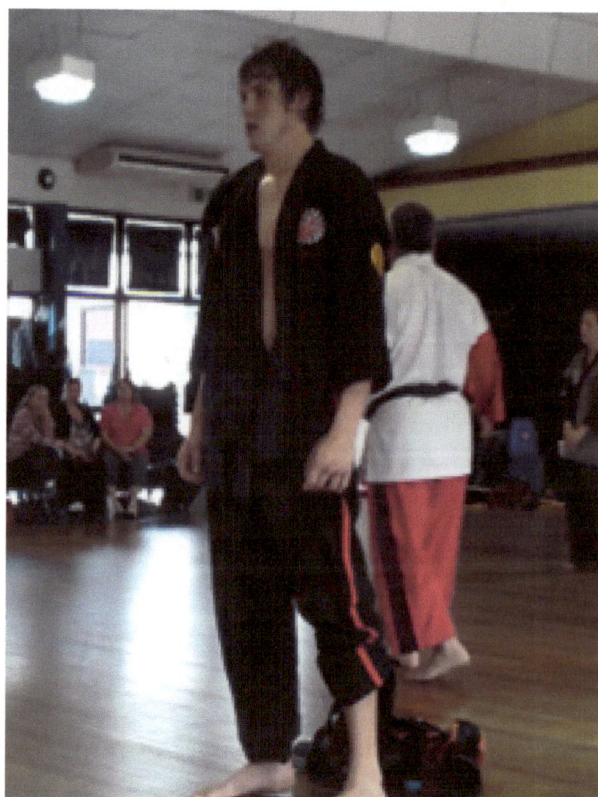

This is me completing my second dan.

The Art and Science of Kundalini
Unveiling the Secrets of Mind, Body, and Energy
by
Scott Butler

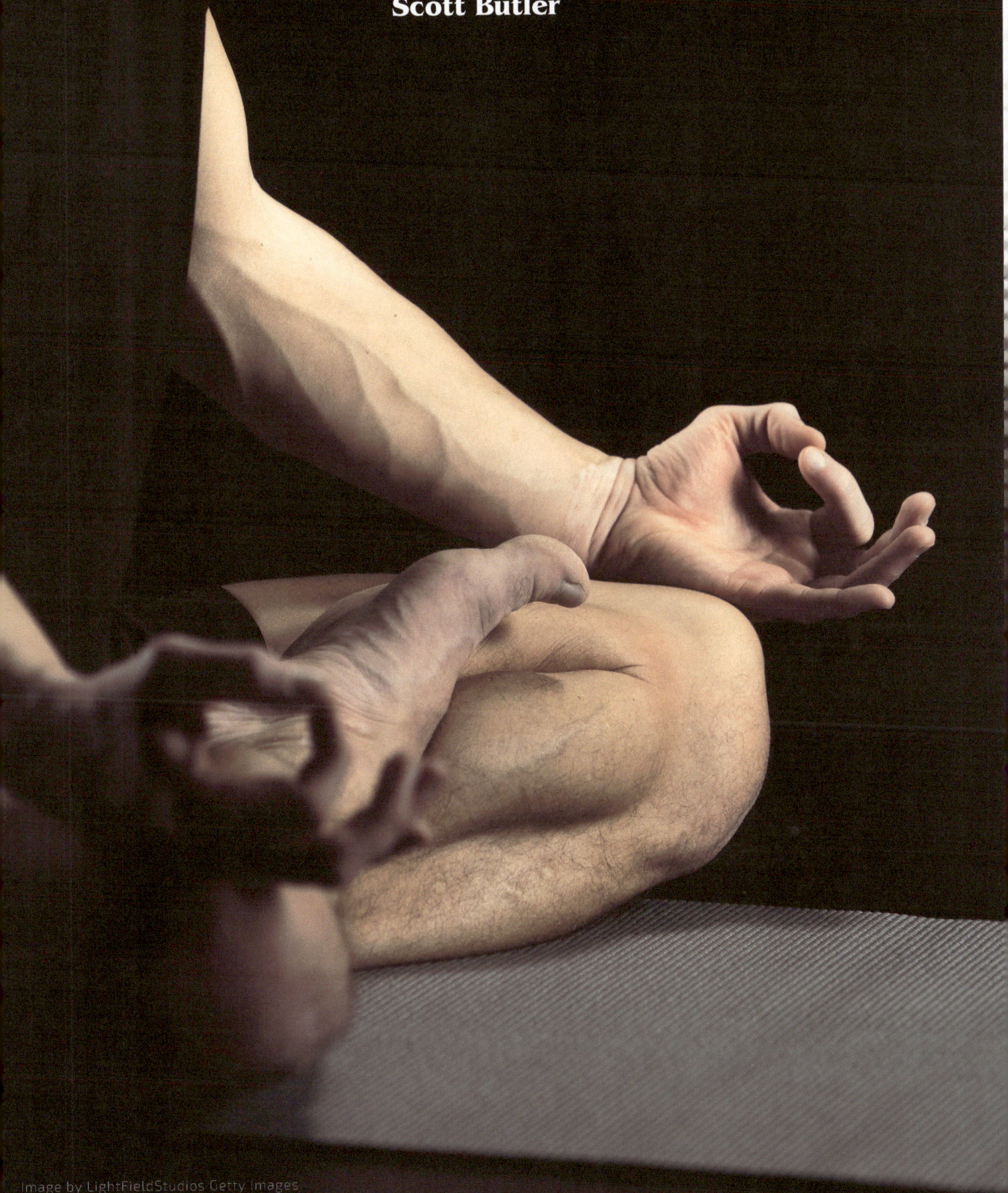

I have been practicing Kundalini for most of my life. It's not merely about yoga; it revolves around breath, energy, health, and power – the power within your body. It encompasses mind-body balance, left and right equilibrium, control, understanding oneself, and comprehending the capabilities of your body.

Take Bruce Lee as an example. Observe him in a fight and contrast it with moments when he isn't engaged. In the latter, he's like anyone else, in a neutral gear. However, during combat, he holds onto energy within his body and manipulates it. This manipulation of energy is what defines Kundalini – being a controlled spring.

Your ability to control this spring is at your discretion. Bruce Lee attained this state through his unique fighting style and extensive training. When you master Kundalini, you grasp the underlying science and can apply it in various ways, from polishing a car to sharpening a knife.

It's not just about hitting a punching bag; it involves every part of your body working together, akin to a stockman's whip. Your body becomes a spring, and Kundalini is intricately tied to your breath, lungs, and the operational condition of your body. It's the distinction between the Flintstone's car and yours, transcending the mere act of using your arm and shoulder – it's a holistic integration of all parts of your being.

Your lungs possess more significance than you realise. Your breathing not only controls your heart but also influences your fatigue, endurance, and overall well-being. Every dedicated cyclist recognises the importance of proper breathing – when done correctly, fatigue is minimised, and one gains control over their heart rate.

In Kundalini, the emphasis is on the pressure held within your lungs and how you utilise it. Picture a balloon that you can squeeze together. The pressure felt during this act is akin to the pressure you can generate within yourself. Mastering the ability to hold on to this pressure takes years. Much like holding your breath, it's about understanding that its energy held within you – physical energy and power, similar to bouncing a ball effortlessly once it's activated.

Generating and holding onto this energy allows you to utilise it effectively, whether it's in physical exercise or martial arts. The fitter you are, the more you can harness this power.

Kundalini is the art of mind-body-spirit harmony. As you progress in knowledge, you remove resistance from your energy system, allowing more power to reach your brain. This enhances cognitive function, focus, and overall physical capabilities.

The practice involves understanding the differences between various martial arts styles and seamlessly switching between them, as they represent different forms of energy flow. Each style is like a different song, with its unique beat and flow. Kundalini, working with energy itself, provides the flexibility to adapt to different styles effortlessly.

The analogy of bouncing a ball illustrates the automatic response once you understand the tempo – your body becomes a coiled spring with controlled, oscillating energy. It's not about imitating a fighting style; it's about feeling and instantly generating the energy that matches the desired style.

Kundalini unlocks your IQ over the long term, offering a myriad of benefits. However, mastering this path requires sacrifices, discipline, and a commitment to a lifelong journey of understanding and expansion.

The practice involves holding the breath and cultivating compassion, engaging every muscle in your body, even those around your eyes and toes. It becomes a level of operation, much like what Bruce Lee demonstrated in his martial arts.

Shaolin Martial arts, while different, shares the concept of held tension. Kundalini pulsates energy continuously back and forth, allowing for a dynamic change in the energy within oneself. It's about defence, countermoves, and flow – a controlled release of stored power.

Understanding the importance of breath, particularly increasing the compression levels within your lungs, is crucial. This, combined with the right muscle coordination, becomes a powerful tool to generate and sustain power. Manipulating this force is akin to being a glass with water, representing an energy mass. Like the water in the glass moves back and forth, you must go with this motion, but you can also manipulate it and change it yourself, allowing you to control the power of your actions and movements.

Bruce Lee serves as an excellent example of someone who knew how to express himself, focusing his intent and holding power like a spring. Observing such mastery is not only amazing but also educational.

Kundalini is about mastering the mind and body, understanding how they work, and utilising that knowledge for personal growth and empowerment.

The Dojo Doctor Answers Your Sticky Training Related Questions

Finding time for training while juggling work, family, and other commitments is challenging. How can I maintain a consistent training schedule without neglecting other aspects of my life?

In the fast-paced rhythm of modern life, finding time for martial arts training can be a Herculean task. Juggling work, family, and other commitments often leaves us feeling like tightrope walkers, desperately seeking balance. Yet, maintaining a consistent training schedule is not only possible but also essential for personal growth and well-being. Here are some practical strategies to help you carve out time for your martial arts journey without neglecting other crucial aspects of your life.

Prioritising and Goal Setting:
The first step in mastering the delicate art of balancing training with life commitments is to set clear priorities and goals. Understand the role martial arts plays in your life—whether it's a form of exercise, stress relief, or personal development. By identifying your priorities, you can allocate time more effectively and ensure that your training aligns with your overall life goals.

Time Management Techniques:
Effective time management is the linchpin of maintaining a consistent training schedule.

Consider implementing time-blocking techniques, where specific blocks of time are dedicated to different activities. Create a weekly schedule that includes designated time slots for work, family, and, of course, martial arts training. Stick to these time blocks as closely as possible to establish a routine that accommodates all facets of your life.

Early Mornings and Late Evenings:
For many individuals, the early morning or late evening hours provide golden opportunities for uninterrupted training sessions. Consider waking up an hour earlier to hit the dojo or practice at home before the day begins. Alternatively, use the quiet hours after everyone else has gone to bed. These time slots not only offer solitude but also set a positive tone for the day or provide a relaxing conclusion to your evening.

Incorporate Family Time:
Integrating martial arts into your family life can be a creative way to spend quality time together while staying committed to your training. Explore family-friendly martial arts activities or encourage your loved ones to join you in light workouts. This not only fosters a supportive environment but also instils a sense of shared accomplishment and well-being.

16

Efficient Training Sessions:

Recognise that the duration of your training sessions doesn't always dictate their effectiveness. Focus on quality rather than quantity. Design workouts that maximise your time and target specific goals. High-intensity interval training (HIIT) and focused, goal-oriented practices can provide substantial benefits in shorter time frames.

Combining Work and Training:

If workable, explore opportunities to integrate martial arts into your work routine. Some workplaces offer fitness facilities or allow employees to take short breaks for physical activity. Incorporating brief stretching or movement exercises during work hours can contribute to your overall fitness and provide a mental refresher.

Open Communication:

Clear communication with your family, employer, and training partners is crucial. Discuss your commitment to martial arts and the importance it holds in your life. By expressing your goals and schedule openly, you create understanding and may even garner support from those around you.

Flexibility and Adaptability:

Life is inherently unpredictable, and rigid schedules can crumble in the face of unexpected challenges. Embrace flexibility and develop the ability to adapt your training routine when necessary. This adaptability ensures that occasional disruptions don't derail your entire plan, allowing you to bounce back quickly and maintain consistency in the long run.

Self-Care and Recovery:

While committing to regular training is essential, so is prioritising self-care and recovery. Over training can lead to burnout and compromise your ability to manage life's demands effectively. Incorporate rest days into your routine, listen to your body, and ensure that your training enhances, rather than hinders, your overall well-being.

Balancing martial arts training with the myriad responsibilities of life is undeniably challenging, but it's a challenge worth embracing. By setting priorities, managing time effectively, and fostering open communication, you can strike a harmonious balance between your training and the other facets of your life. Remember, the journey is as important as the destination, and finding equilibrium is a continuous process that evolves as you grow both as a martial artist and as an individual. Best of luck!

Send your questions to the Dojo Doctor - at info@MartialArtsMagazineAustralia

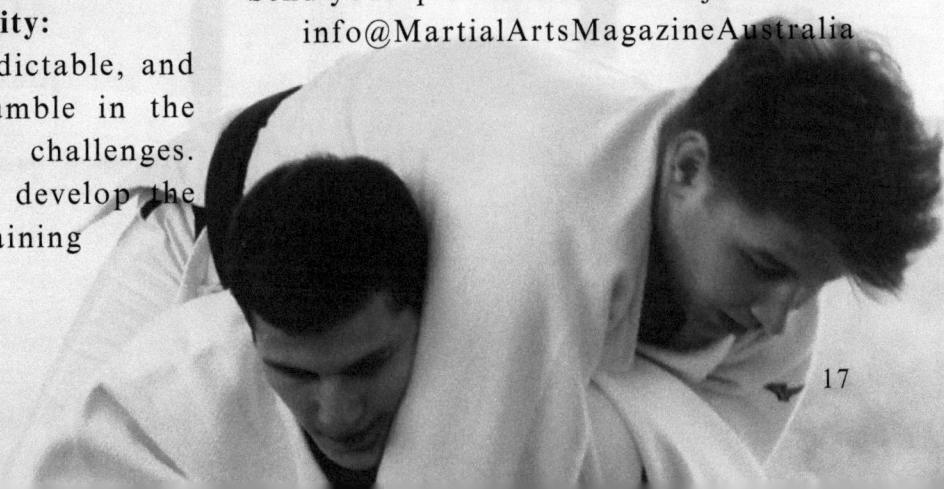

I get extremely nervous before competitions, and it is affecting my performance. Do you have any tips for managing pre-competition stress and staying focused?

Competing in martial arts can be a thrilling and rewarding experience, but the anxiety that precedes competitions is a common hurdle many practitioners face. Pre-competition nervousness can significantly impact performance, hindering the ability to showcase one's skills effectively.

Before exploring coping strategies, it's essential to recognise that feeling nervous before a competition is entirely normal. In fact, a certain level of nervousness can be beneficial, as it signifies a heightened state of alertness and readiness. The key is to manage these nerves in a way that enhances performance rather than detracts from it.

Mental Preparation:

Adequate mental preparation is fundamental in managing pre-competition stress. Visualisation techniques can be powerful tools to create a mental image of success. Spend time mentally rehearsing your techniques, imagining yourself executing flawless moves with precision. This not only reinforces muscle memory, but also instils a sense of confidence in your abilities.

Breathing Exercises:

Controlled breathing is a proven method of managing stress and anxiety. Implement deep breathing exercises, focusing on slow inhalations and exhalations. Practice diaphragmatic breathing to calm the nervous system and centre your mind. Incorporate these exercises into your pre-competition routine to establish a sense of 'tranquillity'.

Progressive Muscle Relaxation:

Tension often accompanies nervousness, leading to physical tightness and diminished performance. Progressive Muscle Relaxation (PMR) is a technique where you systematically tense and then release each muscle group in your body. This process helps alleviate physical tension, promoting a state of relaxation. Practice PMR during your warm-up or in the moments leading up to your competition.

Establish a Routine:

Create a pre-competition routine that encompasses both physical and mental aspects. Engage in familiar warm-up exercises and rituals that bring a sense of normalcy to the environment. Establishing a routine signals to your brain that it's time to transition into competition mode, minimising the impact of anxiety.

Positive Affirmations:

The power of positive affirmations should not be underestimated. Develop a set of affirmations that resonate with you and focus on your strengths and capabilities. Repeat these affirmations before and during the competition to shift your mindset from anxiety to empowerment.

Focus on the Process:

Redirect your attention from the potential outcomes of the competition to the process itself. Concentrate on executing each technique flawlessly, staying present in the moment. By shifting your focus to the task at hand, you mitigate the overwhelming pressure associated with the end result.

Pre-Competition Routine:

Craft a pre-competition routine that includes activities you find calming and enjoyable. Whether it's listening to music, engaging in light stretching, or reading a motivational quote, these rituals can serve as comforting anchors in the midst of pre-competition nerves.

Utilise Arousal Control:

Understand the concept of arousal control, which involves regulating the level of excitement and energy before a competition. Experiment with techniques to either increase or decrease arousal based on your individual needs. Some may benefit from energetic activities to raise arousal, while others might find calm activities more effective.

Seek Professional Guidance:

If pre-competition anxiety becomes overwhelming and persistent, consider seeking guidance from a sports psychologist or mental performance coach. These professionals specialise in helping athletes develop coping strategies, manage stress, and optimise their mental state for peak performance.

Learn from Experience:

Each competition provides an opportunity to learn more about yourself and your reactions to stress. After each event, reflect on your experiences—what worked, what didn't, and how you can improve your pre-competition routine. This reflective practice contributes to ongoing personal growth and enhanced performance in future competitions.

Pre-competition stress is a shared experience among martial artists, but with the right strategies, it can be managed effectively. By incorporating mental preparation, breathing exercises, relaxation techniques, and positive affirmations into your routine, you can transform pre-competition nerves into a source of strength and focus. Remember, the journey to mastering pre-competition jitters is as individual as your martial arts practice, and finding the right combination of strategies may require some experimentation. With perseverance and a proactive mindset, you can step onto the competition mat with confidence, ready to showcase your skills and embrace the thrill of the martial arts journey. Best of Luck!

Peanut Butter Banana Protein Smoothie

This smoothie provides a good balance of protein, healthy fats, fibre, potassium and other nutrients to help rebuild muscles, restore energy levels and hydrate. The peanut butter and protein powder offer muscle-building amino acids while the banana, flaxseed and honey provide quick carbohydrates to replenish glycogen after an intense workout. Adjust ingredients to suit your own nutritional needs and taste preferences.

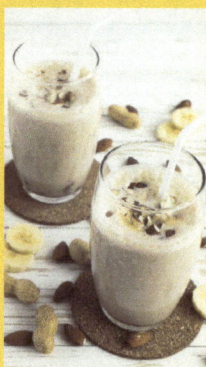

Ingredients:
1 banana, frozen
1 cup milk of choice (dairy, almond, soy, etc.)
2 tablespoons peanut butter
2 tablespoons protein powder
1 tablespoon ground flaxseed
1 tablespoon honey
Ice cubes (optional)

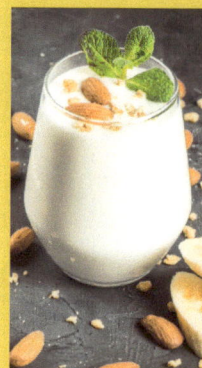

Directions:
1. Add the frozen banana, milk, peanut butter, protein powder, flaxseed, and honey to a high-powered blender.
2. Blend until smooth and creamy. If too thick, add a few ice cubes to reach desired consistency.
3. Pour into a glass and enjoy after your training session.

AIKIDO ADVENTURES IN VIENNA

by

Attila Halasz

It was 1995 when I, a young lad from Australia, stepped into the bustling city of Vienna, Austria. Eager to explore the local martial arts scene, I checked the phone book and confirmed my attendance at a Vienna-style (Aikikai) Aikido dojo, even though it wasn't my usual Australian Shin Sen Dojo style.

Walking into a foreign dojo is always a thrill!

After changing into my gi, I noticed three fellow black belts – two female and a male Aikidoka – and an intriguing figure, another odd-looking black belt. Clad in black pants and a jacket adorned with a red Ninjutsu symbol, he stood out without a hakama.

The fourth-degree black belt teacher, around fifty and visibly tired from a day's work, led the class through basic drills. The class, consisting of 13 practitioners, felt ordinary and uninspiring, until an unexpected turn of events unfolded.

The ninja, seemingly polite up to this point, stood up and announced, that as part of his black belt experience, he came to challenge the Sensei on the mat. The challenge was set: the one who gets pinned loses.

Excitement filled the air! I sat cross-legged, anticipating the upcoming challenges. "Oh, this is great," I said.

The first fight was taken by a female Aikidoist. The ninja attacked with a mild forward strike, which she countered with a large turn, deeply entering around the strike. Half way through her technique, the ninja suddenly changed position as if he expected the irimi nage, struck towards her face and took her down with a sudden hip throw. Locked her with his knees until she tapped out. His stealth was incredibly clever!

Next up was the male black belt, but by now, the polite ninja facade all but disappeared. After a front kick and middle body punch, he took down the Aikidoist with a leg sweep and struck his head. He too tapped out. The ninja was fast and determined to get to the Sensei.

The last female black belt was already startled before the fight. The ninja spent an easy few seconds to take her down.

There was a surprised silence. The ninja looked at me, not sure about my status.

According to the dojo specific challenge, the Sensei had to be next.

He sat under the photo of O Sensei, calm and motionless. One could tell that his mind was elsewhere, maybe other worries, not particularly about fighting a ninja on a Wednesday night. I looked at him with a question mark. Our eyes locked. I read his intention and knew what to do. He just made me a student of this dojo. I bowed to the ninja and walked out onto the mat.

The entire class looked on, some of them smiling. It was their turn to be excited by the visiting Australian.

I faced the approaching ninja calmly. He thought I would be defensive, like the others before me. However, I suddenly attacked him with a front kick and a temple strike right after. This momentum made him step back. When he lifted his arm to block my head strike, there was the perfect opportunity for me for the ikkyo ura, inside stepping joint lock, done fast with weight kept underside. This time the ninja was brought down on the floor and I put on a classic arm pin until he tapped out. My home dojo was budo focused, using ki power. Always considering the moment of life and death.

The challenge and the class were over. As a lovely gesture, the group, including the Sensei, were clapping.

The ninja bowed, then made a farewell speech that although he won three fights, in the end he was defeated and he has learnt that Aikido is a force to be reckoned with and this, he will take back to his dojo and his own sensei.

Afterwards we all went out for drinks and I can tell you, Vienna is expensive, but somehow I ended up not paying for any of my drinks. What a great night it was!

The next day, I packed up my gear and went on by train, this time to face an even greater challenge in a French aikido camp. But that's another story.

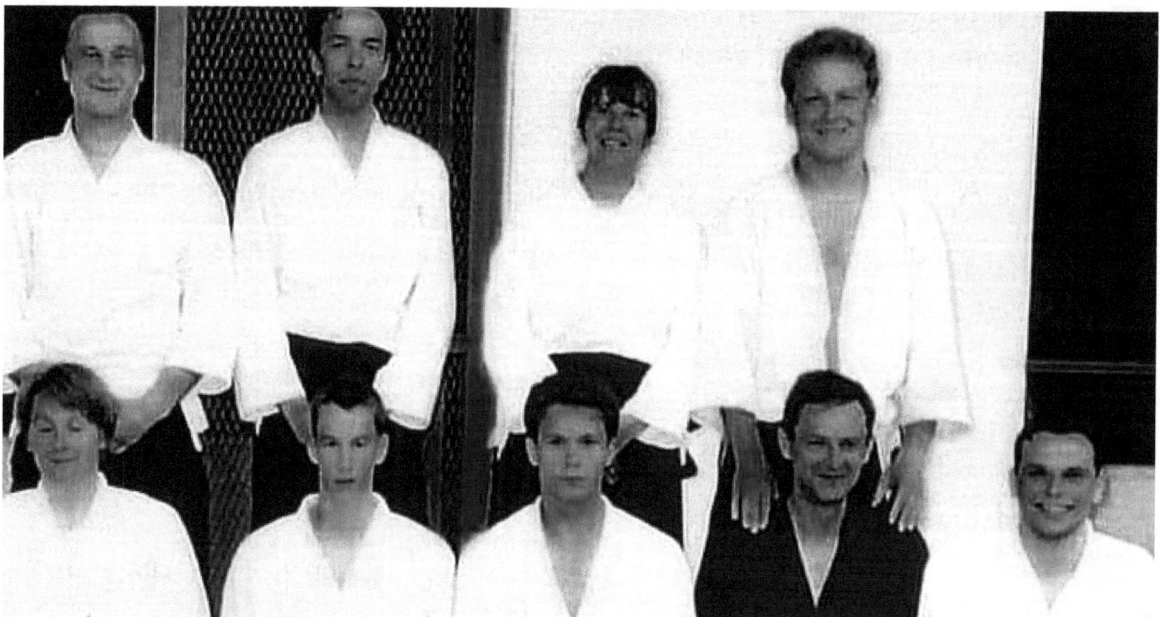

The Vienna Aikikai dojo, 1995. I'm standing with the visiting ninja kneeling in front.

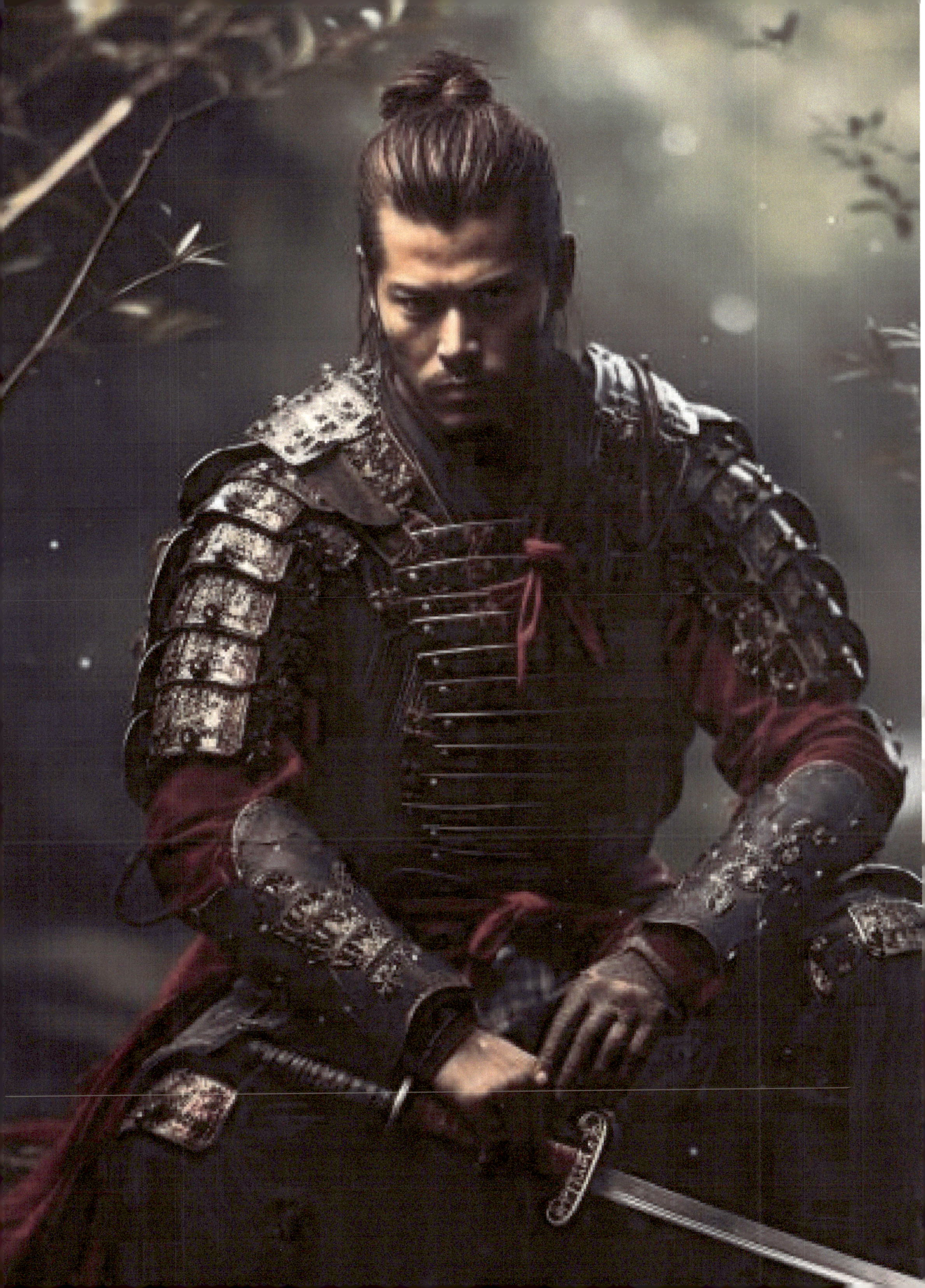

Is it Possible to be a Samurai in Modern Day Australia?

by Tim Webster

Samurai: *The fearless warrior of old Japan. Sword in hand, battling through charging enemies, willing to sacrifice himself for his lord.*

Those of us who study any traditional Japanese martial art, have likely been told about Samurai, and those who don't will still know plenty from all the movies and books created about them.

The Samurai are heavily associated with the warrior's code, Bushido, which is literally - *The Way of the Warrior.* Bushido is a set of values dealing with virtuous attitudes and strengths.

Samurai lived a life of service to their clan and lord. The actual word Samurai 侍 means – To Serve.

But to serve what? What does that mean?

To really understand what this means, we have to become familiar with the concept of *Giri.* Giri is at the heart of what it means to serve, to be Samurai.

Giri is duty, it is obligation, it is loyalty. It is the most powerful part of Bushido.

A duty not just to an individual, but to society itself. It is a willing obligation to do what is right and uphold a high moral standard.

Giri is something that people take pride in.

Giri is unconditional, no credit is sought after or is required.

Where martial arts in Japan are concerned, Giri is about training to the best of your ability and defeating the opponent as efficiently as possible with honour. It is also about following your teacher with devotion and loyalty, as they have done for their teacher before.

Having something like this to work towards gives us a path to follow.

My teacher, SeiShihan Goho, is turning 90 this year and he is still training and teaching at his Dojo every week. He is a great example of Giri and a model of what to live by, physically and mentally. He loyally followed his teacher, Grandmaster Kimura, right up until the end of his teacher's life. When Grandmaster Kimura passed away, his son, SeiShihan Toru Kimura, became the Inheritor to the style in Nagoya, Japan, and we now follow him loyally.

Giri is a huge part of all Japanese martial arts, but it is also very present in other Japanese ways like Chado(tea-cermony), Shodo (Calligraphy), and others. It is also a big part of Japanese culture and society still today.

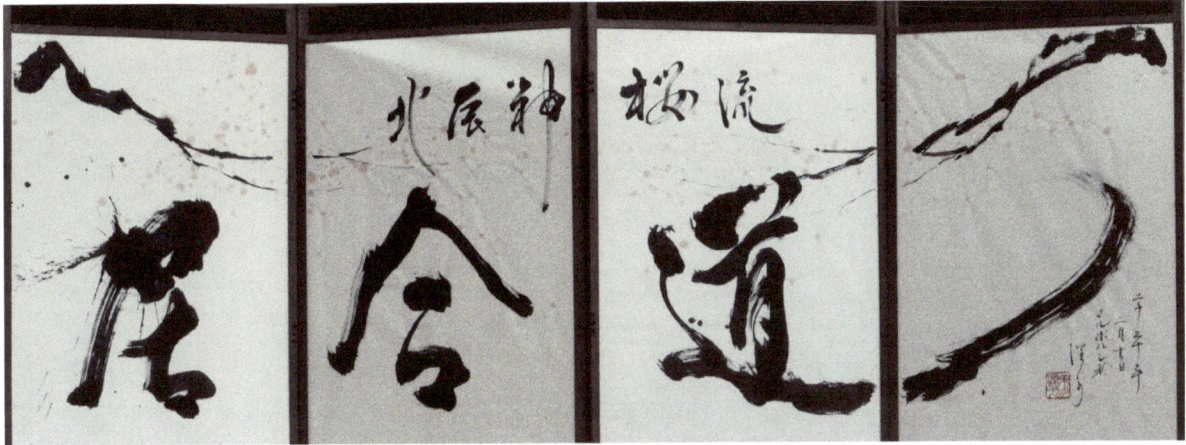

Iaido Kanji Calligraphy

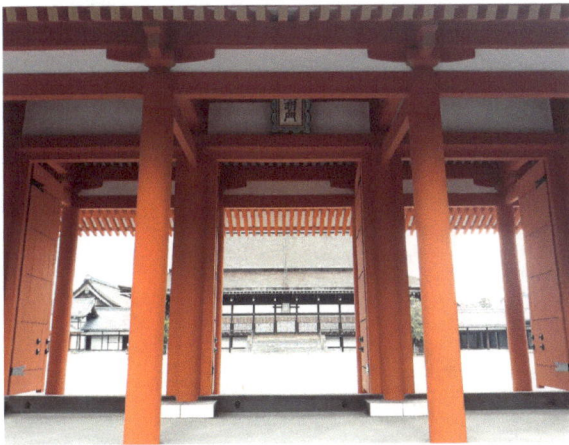

Gate to old Emperor's Palace Kyoto

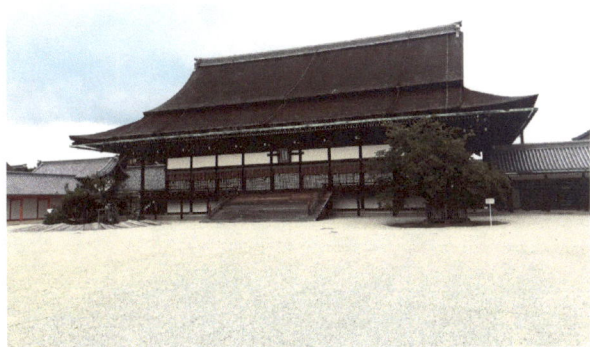

Kyoto old Emperor's Palace

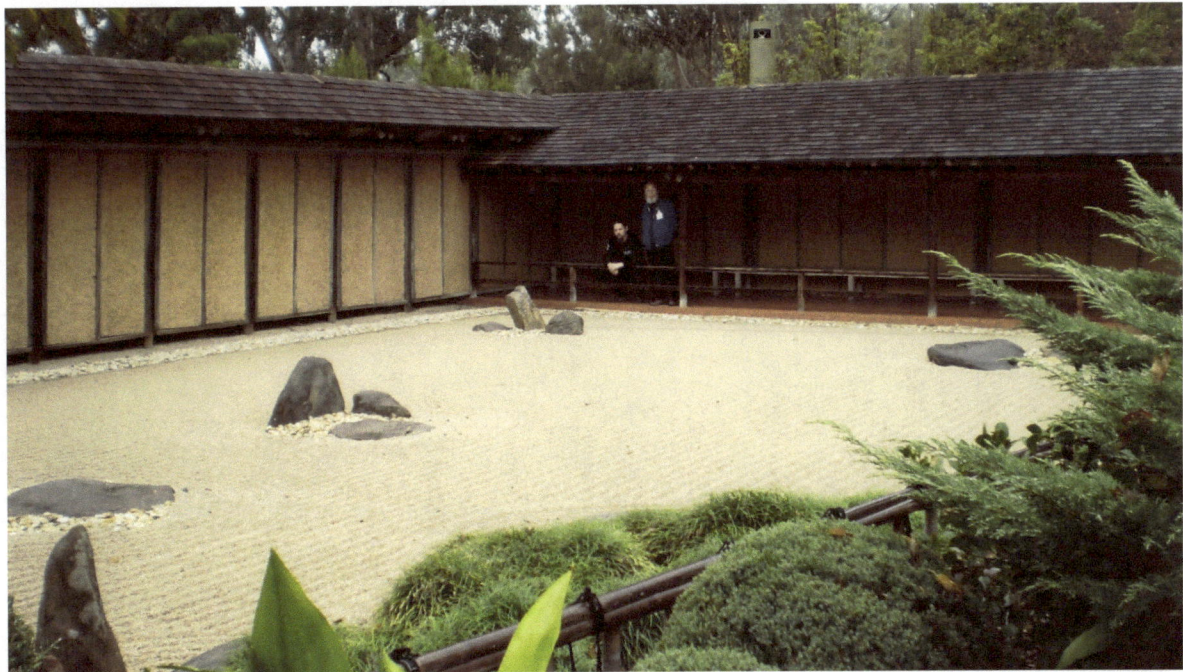

Images by Tim Webster

Sensei Tim with SeiShihan Goho at Zen Garden

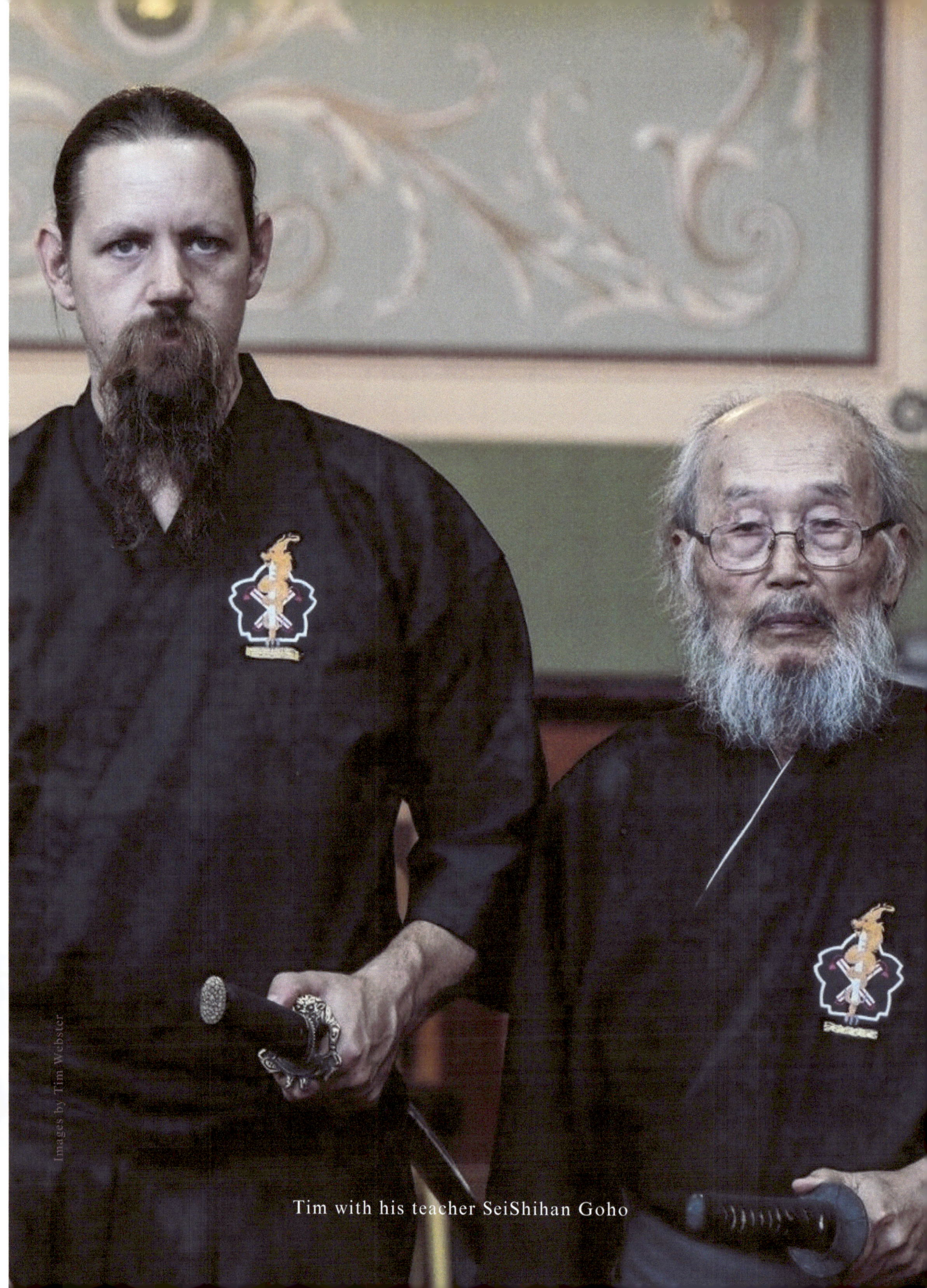
Tim with his teacher SeiShihan Goho

Giri underpins general day to day activity in Japan. Work obligations performed to the best of an individual's ability, trains and road crossings politely and efficiently dealt with in a respectful way. It is also doing the right thing and standing up for what is just, and defending that to the end.

What does all that have to do with us Aussies?

In Australia, we are happy cooking a BBQ, having a beer and watching the footy, while complaining about work or the bloody government. But the concept of Giri is active in modern day Australia. It is in our martial arts of course, but it is also in our society.

The Aussie idea of "Sticking up for your mate" or "A Fair go" or "Mateship" are all a form of Giri.

If you have ever gone to defend someone who is being threatened, if you have helped a stranger, if you have donated to charity or if you have given without expecting something in return, then that is Giri.

Those of us who train in a form of martial arts in Australia, we know we train hard. We train to defeat the opponent as quickly and efficiently as possible. We train to the best of our abilities, and we try to improve and do better. We learn from our Sensei and we are loyal and devoted to them.

However, most people today start training in martial arts because they want to get something out if it. That's why we do most things.

We want to learn to defend ourselves, we want to get fit, we want our children to gain some self-confidence or discipline.

These are all good reasons, but they are us wanting to get something out of it for ourselves.

To look at things with Giri in mind we should start to shift from, "what can we get out of it for us?" to "what can we put into it? What we can give back to it?" This way, we can start to view things through the eyes of a Samurai.

So whether we are seasoned instructors with decades of martial arts experience, or new students busily learning and training as much as we can, or even someone who is just now thinking about taking up a form of martial arts, there is something inside this idea that we can all try to embrace.

This idea of Samurai has nothing to do with if you train using a sword or not. The sword is a symbol, just like it was to the Samurai in the days of old.

Whether we train Karate, Aikido, BJJ, MMA, Muay Thai or any other art, we should train to the best of our ability, learn to face and defeat our opponent as efficiently as possible and do it with honour.

We should also, when possible, learn to avoid the unnecessary spilling of blood. You can avoid confrontation by not drawing your sword and cutting them down, or not using the most severe technique in your set of abilities.

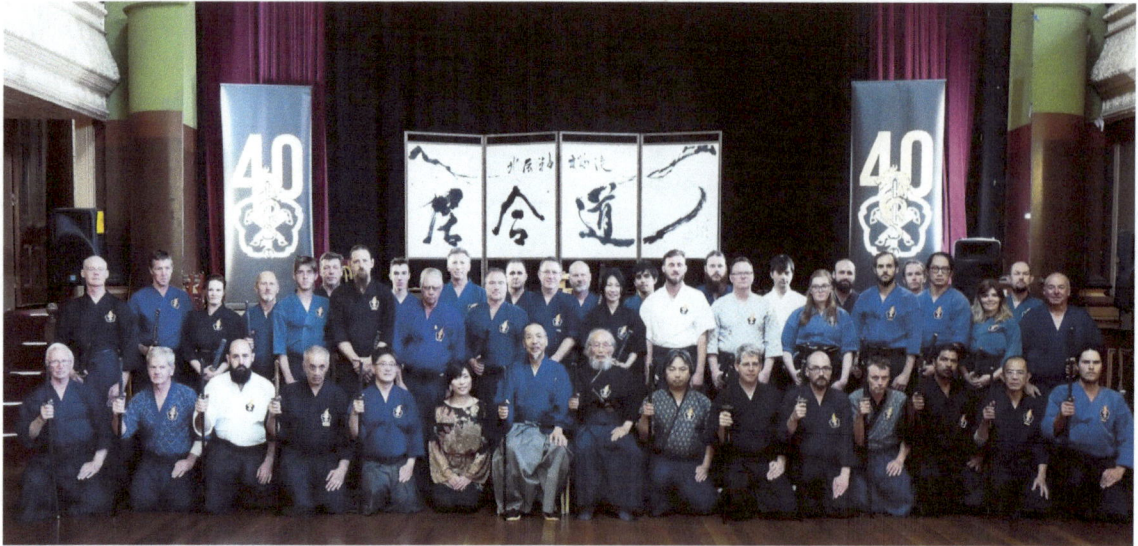

40th Anniversary of HSR Iaido in Australia Melbourne 2020

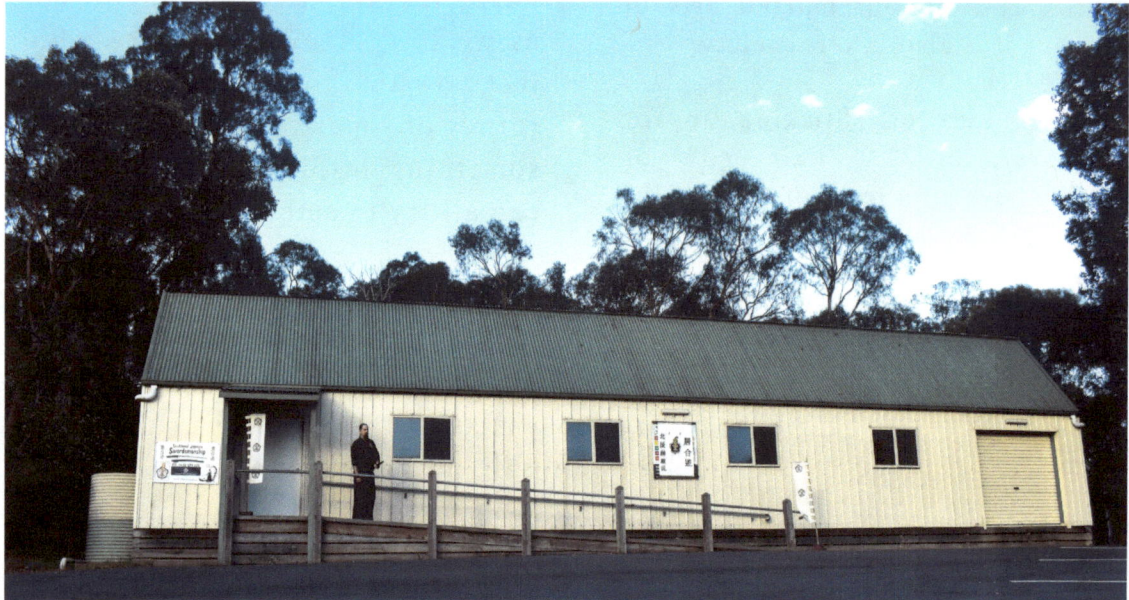

Tim at his Dojo on the hill in Eltham, Melbourne

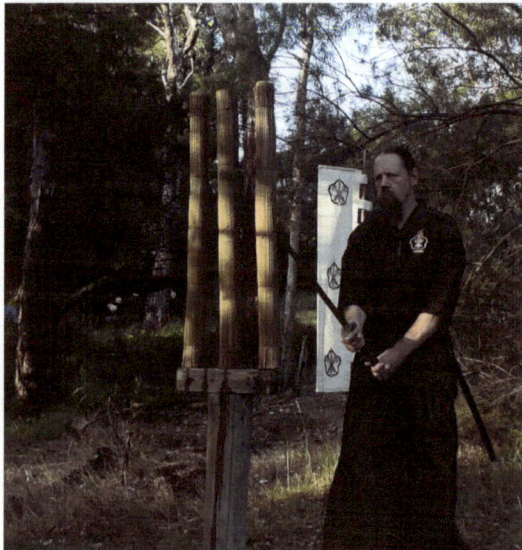

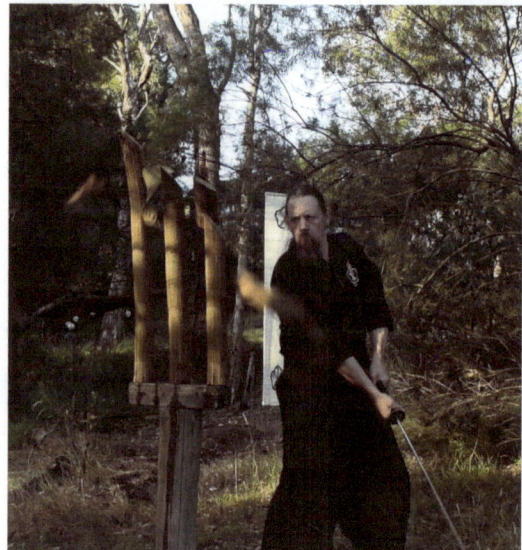

Tameshigiri 1 & 2

By avoiding a confrontation with someone, we can avoid unnecessary bloodshed. This is also a practice of Giri.

My Master SeiShihan Goho has said many times, "If everyone could think this way, we would have peace in the world."

Keeping this in mind, the more obscure ideas can come into focus. We can let our misconceptions fall away and see what Samurai really means beyond the romance of the movie screen. We can live without fear and let our willing obligation show us the true path forward. We can serve others, we can live with honour.

To think like a Samurai, you have to have a deep understanding of Giri.
If you embrace Giri, then all the other concepts that are in Bushido, like loyalty, honour, respect, honesty, and courage will happen naturally.

Whether it is standing in the ring ready for the bell, or standing up to a bully who is out in the street, whether it is having to overcome an injury in training, or having to overcome a difficulty in family life, whether it is stepping onto the mat to face an opponent, or stepping out of your front door to face the world, this is Giri.

Chances are that if you are reading this article, you can probably see how many of these ideas apply to you already. Perhaps you are Samurai.

Maybe many of us already are Samurai, just in ways that we may not have realised.

But that is the special and important part. We do it unconditionally, like a parent dedicating their lives to their children. We do it without expecting something in return.

Then, once we understand this, it is our duty to try to teach others what it means.

So, to answer the question from the beginning, yes, I think it is possible to be a Samurai in modern day Australia. We just have to have a true understanding of GIRI.

We definitely shouldn't go around thinking we are Samurai, but we should do our best to try to think like Samurai

We should never say that we are Samurai, we should just do our best to act like Samurai.

So then, the next question is how can we be better Samurai?

You, the person reading this now, has the opportunity and the task, as was the case with Samurai of the past, to improve.

- Try to do better in training.

- Try to do better in life.

The sword is a symbol, to be sworn on as an instrument of justice, always carried by Samurai.

In modern day Australia, we can't walk around outside carrying a sword in our hand or belt.

But we can walk around outside carrying our sword in our heart and mind.

Sensei Tim Webster is a 6th Dan Instructor in the traditional Japanese swordsmanship style - Hokushin Shinoh Ryu Iai-Do, under Master SeiShihan Goho Wonho Chong and Kaicho Suseki Shihan Takeo Matsunami Chong.

Sensei Tim is also a long term student of Sensei Herve Vengtasamy at Lion Heart Mixed Martial Arts in Bundoora, studying in other Japanese arts such as Karate and Aikido.

Sensei Tim runs KenDo-Kan, a small swordsmanship dojo in Eltham, Melbourne.

Hokushin Shinoh Ryu Iaido Swordsmanship has International Dojos across Australia and New Zealand.

For more Info visit – www.hokushin.com.au or the Hokushin Shinoh Ryu Facebook pages in Adelaide, Melbourne, Bendigo & Canberra.

Image
Sengakuji Temple, Japan, gravesite to the famous 47 Ronin Samurai

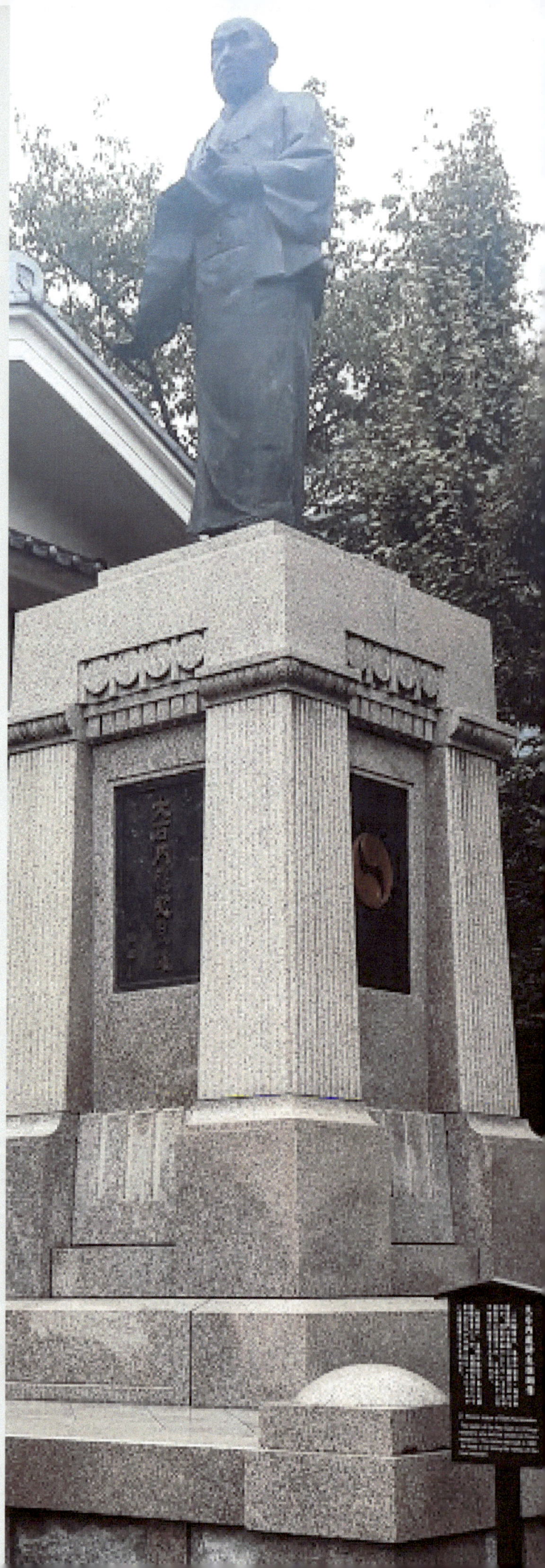

Image Tim Webster

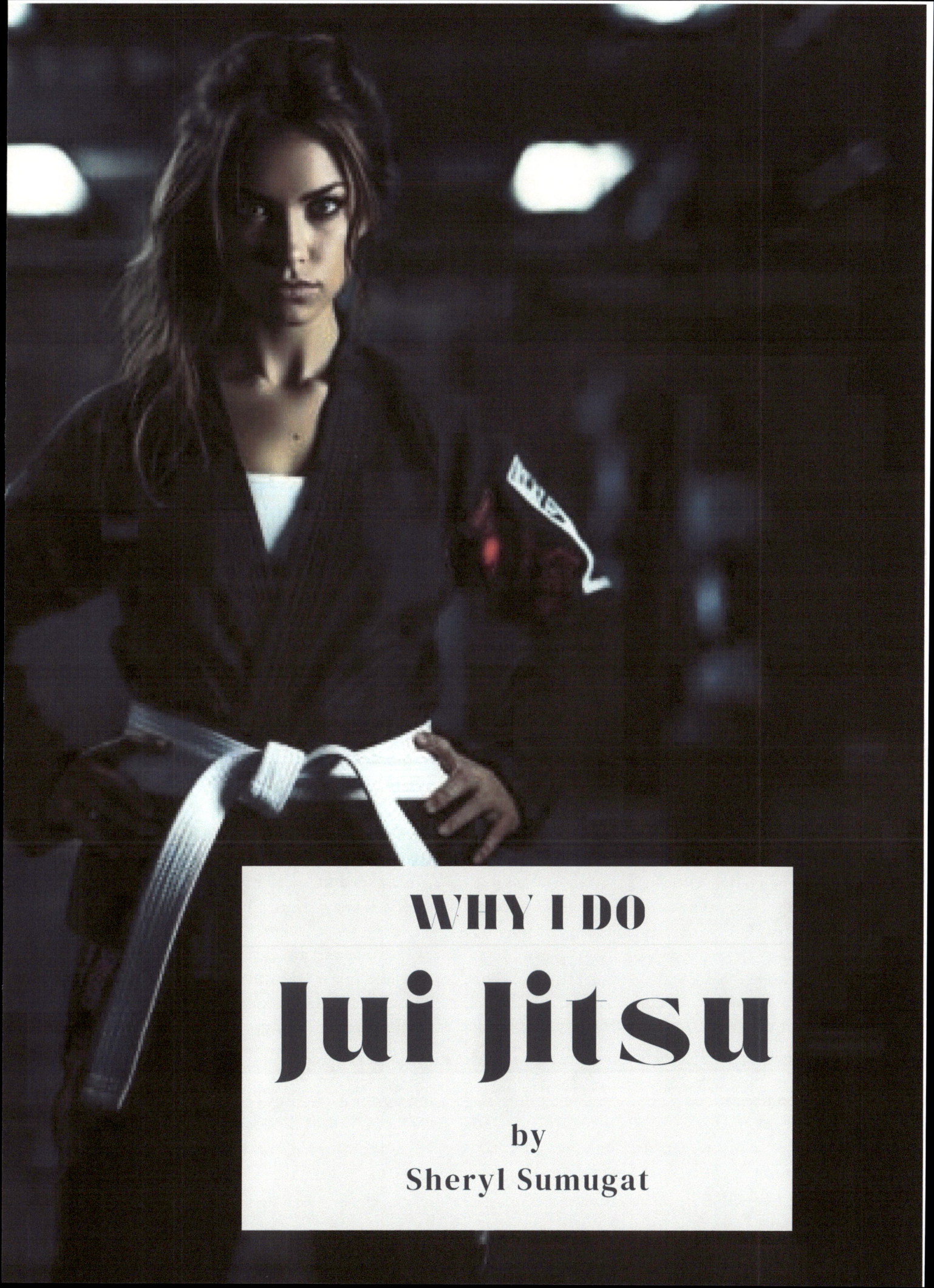

WHY I DO
Jui Jitsu

by

Sheryl Sumugat

I took off my Gi and breathed a sigh of relief. I had only been doing Jiu Jitsu for less than a month. I still hadn't gotten used to being pinned on the mat. The session was finally over, and I didn't feel any wiser. The woman sitting across from me noticed the frustration on my face. Unlike me, she had been doing it for years. Small talk ensued. I told her some days my mind just couldn't grasp the techniques, and she said, "But you enjoy it, right?"

My husband introduced me to Jiu Jitsu. It's the love of his life. As a joke, I had a shirt made for him that says, "I love my family...but not as much as Jiujitsu." I've always found it boring and too technical. Jiu Jitsu is not a spectator sport, unlike boxing or Muay Thai. It took me a long time to finally give it a go, and it wasn't because of him. I bet some of my friends think I'm doing Jiu Jitsu to impress him or because he had finally convinced me to. He never did.

I was doom scrolling when I came across a triggering article. The home my husband and I work so hard to build is safe and happy, but I used to live in one where I had to walk on eggshells. Although it was a long time ago, it went on for several years. Riddled with unprocessed trauma, I can get triggered by the simplest things. And when I do, I freeze. The few times my father almost hit me, I never tried to run or fight. I just froze like a punching bag, waiting to be annihilated. It got so bad I contemplated suicide at one point. It went on for a long time until my dad got cancer. He did change, and the bond was repaired, but the damage was done.

It's never easy revealing a painful past and I do not enjoy talking negatively about my dad, but it is what it is. The main reason I put on a gi and get on the mat is because I am still that vulnerable young person. I realised I had been dealing with it all through repression. The past can creep up on us when we least expect it. When it does, I want to be prepared. I want to be able to do something other than freeze.

I still haven't gotten to where I consider Jiujitsu to be a hobby. To me, it's mandatory like P.E., and I was never good at it. When the nice lady asked if I enjoyed it, I replied, "Nah." I don't enjoy it. I'd much rather paint or do some gardening. She then asked, "Then why do you do it?" I simply replied, "Because it's a good skill to learn." I couldn't tell her that it's because the young version of me who was stuck in an abusive home still needs to be saved. **I showed up at least once a week at the gym despite not having enough sleep for the young girl that felt helpless.**

Someday it will get easier, and I will start enjoying it as much as the lady I was talking to. Someday I will do it because it's fun. In the meantime, it's because it's part of my healing, even if it's hard and uncomfortable. You can't freeze when you're about to get choked. To survive, movement is vital but so is breathing and taking a moment to think and not just react out of fear or impulse. This is what Jiu Jitsu has taught me. It is intense yet calming. It is a practice of staying calm in the face of danger. To a traumatized brain like mine, it is medication without its negative side effects. And as I type in these thoughts, I came into the realization that I am starting to love it.

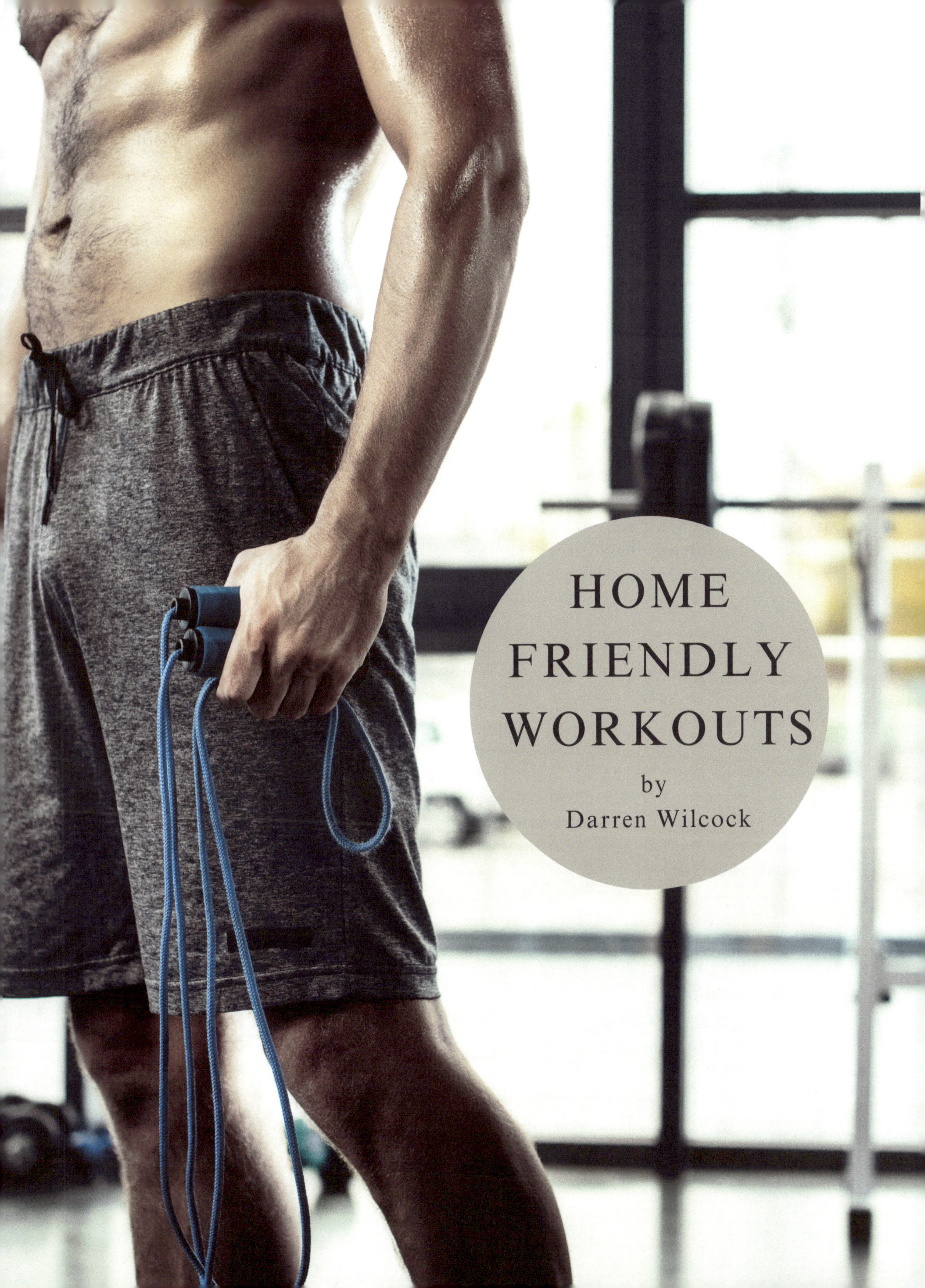

HOME FRIENDLY WORKOUTS

by

Darren Wilcock

The world was emerging from a pandemic that confined most of us within the four walls of home, cutting us off from our regular escapes like going to the gym or dojo. For me, like so many others, this absence left a massive void in my life.

You see, training and going to the gym is my lifeline, connecting me with likeminded people who share a passion for chosen physical pursuits. We build lasting bonds that span countries. So when the lockdowns hit, I turned to social media to get my much-needed fix, joining groups covering the martial arts and combat sports I practice. Some simply discussed famous martial artists and combat athletes, but others shared training routines and asked for tips on staying fit at home.

It became clear some people still struggled with home workouts, lacking equipment or space to train properly alone. As someone from the fitness industry, I saw even as things reopened, gyms struggled to recover. So I decided to provide simple yet effective home workouts using little or no equipment, substituting household items when needed.

The following workouts can help you maintain or build fitness right from your living room. All you need is some determination!

Routine 1-level beginner
Equipment skipping rope.

Move through the skipping and exercises without stopping. If you can't skip, you can purchase skipping rope handles with a small amount of rope on and then a light weight to simulate the feeling of the skipping rope so all you have to do is count your jumps.

Remember, a skipping rope is only a few millimetres thick, so this is as high as you need to jump. If you are weak at push ups, you can use a regression and do them on your knees, but to get better at them I would try to do the 1,2 & 3 in a full push up position if possible. Only using the regression as needed:

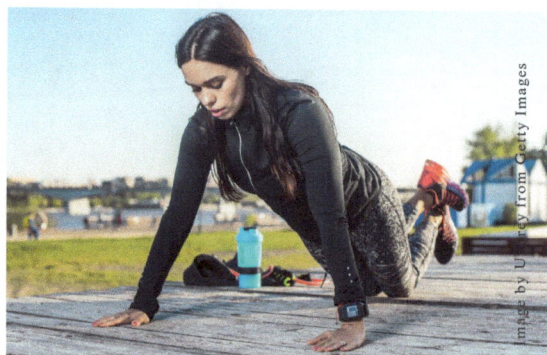

100 revolutions of skipping rope (slow)
100 revolutions of skipping rope (fast)
1 push up, 1 crunch, 1 squat.
80 revolutions of skipping rope (slow)
80 revolutions of skipping rope (fast)
2 push ups, 2 crunch, 2 squats.
60 revolutions of skipping rope (slow)
60 revolutions of skipping rope (fast)
3 push ups, 3 crunch, 3 squats
40 revolutions of skipping rope (slow)
40 revolutions of skipping rope (fast)
4 push ups, 4 crunch, 4 squats
20 revolutions of skipping rope (slow)
20 revolutions of skipping rope (fast)
5 push ups, 5 crunch, 5 squats
10 revolutions of skipping rope (slow)
10 revolutions of skipping rope (fast)
6 push ups, 6 crunch, 6 squats

That's a very basic workout and like I said it's aimed at a beginner, moving on from that to someone with more fitness you can do a similar thing such as:

100 revolutions of skipping rope (slow)
100 revolutions of skipping rope (fast)
1 push up, 1 crunch, 1 squat.
90 revolutions of skipping rope (slow)
90 revolutions of skipping rope (fast)
2 push ups, 2 crunch, 2 squats.
80 revolutions of skipping rope (slow)
80 revolutions of skipping rope (fast)
3 push ups, 3 crunch, 3squats,
70 revolutions of skipping rope (slow)
70 revolutions of skipping rope (fast)
4 push ups, 4 crunch, 4 squats,
60 revolutions of skipping rope (slow)
60 revolutions of skipping rope (fast)
5 push ups, 5crunch, 5 squats
50 revolutions of skipping rope (slow)
50 revolutions of skipping rope (fast)
6 push ups ,6 crunch, 6 squats
40 revolutions of skipping rope (slow)
40 revolutions of skipping rope (fast)
7 push ups, 7 crunch, 7 squats
30 revolutions of skipping rope (slow)
30 revolutions of skipping rope (fast)
8 push ups, 8 crunch, 8 squats,
20 revolutions of skipping rope (slow)
20 revolutions of skipping rope (fast)
9 push ups, 9 crunch, 9 squats
10 revolutions of skipping rope (slow)
10 revolutions of skipping rope (fast)
10 push ups, 10 crunch, 10 squats.

If you want something a little more challenging, use the above skipping matrix 100 slow, 100 fast, going down in tens but substitute the push ups for burpees, crunch can be a weighted crunch as can the squat or change that to a jump squat or even a tuck jump. If you are at home and don't have any weights, that's ok, improvise. You could use a 5kg bag of potatoes, just hold it on your chest and do the crunch or squat.

For some people out there, this could be easy and if that's the case, use these routines as a warmup before doing some shadow boxing rounds or going through a kata, or even just to get you ready for some stretching.

These are just some ideas to keep you on track if you can't make it to the gym, or you're wanting to do some extra work to improve your overall fitness. It's a quick little workout that should only take around 20 minutes.

Skipping is an excellent cardiovascular exercise that you will notice the benefits of in a short time if done consistently. You could do one of these workouts 2/3 times a week as well as your normal martial arts class and watch your fitness improve.

Obviously get clearance from a doctor before starting exercising, especially if you haven't done anything physical in sometime, or like me you're on the wrong side of 50 (hahaha).

Remember, if you want to see results, consistency is key. Stick with it! Put a red mark on a calendar on the days you train or keep an exercise diary. These will help you stay consistent.

If you like the above options of workout or you're looking for something more specific, training for a particular body part let me know and maybe I could help you out. But for now, stay strong, stay fit and stay healthy. OOOOOOOOOSH!

Darren Wilcock is a personal trainer and can be contacted at:
fitnesspotentialunleashed@gmail.com

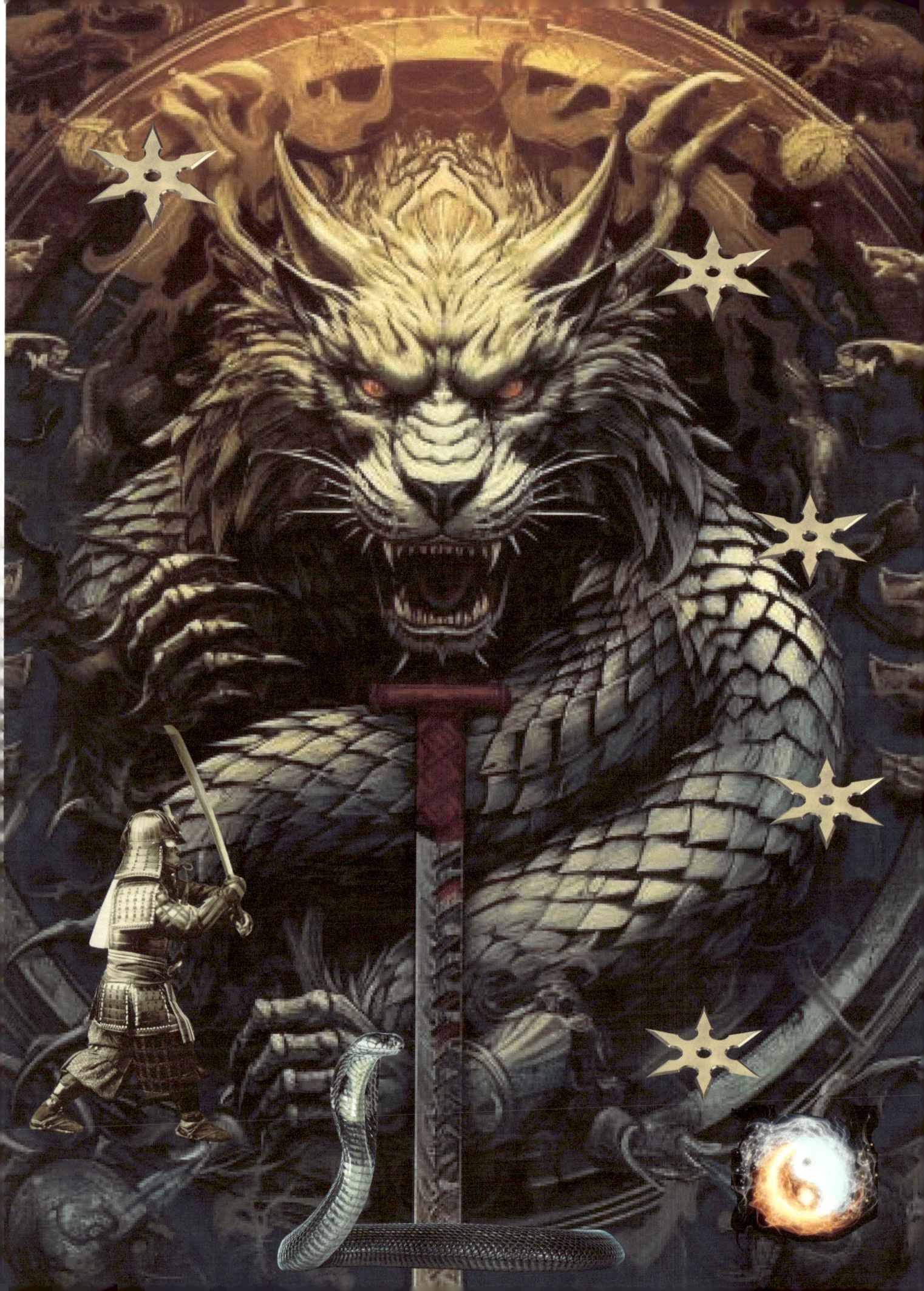

SYMBOLISM IN MARTIAL ARTS

by

Hahn O'Dowd

Martial arts are deeply rooted in history, tradition, and cultural meaning. Symbolism plays an integral role in many styles of martial arts across the world. From the iconic yin and yang symbol to animal representations and weapons, symbols are incorporated into training, uniforms, philosophy and more. These symbols often have layered meanings that tell us about the origins and beliefs behind martial art practices.

The dragon is one of the most ubiquitous symbols in Chinese martial arts like Kung Fu. The dragon represents power, strength, and excellence. It is seen as a spiritual and noble creature that protects the innocent. In Kung Fu, the dragon is celebrated through dragon dances, regalia, and even styles like "dragon claw." Dragon symbols inspire students to channel qualities like courage and leadership. The dragon's fluid, flexible movements are also an ideal for Kung Fu practitioners to emulate. Even Bruce Lee chose the dragon to represent his personal philosophy of Jeet Kune Do, representing his desire to be formless and adaptable.

The classic Yin Yang symbol permeates Eastern philosophy and martial arts. The intertwined black and white halves represent complementary opposites: dark-light, fire-water, masculine-feminine.

The symbol teaches an appreciation of balance and harmony between seeming contradictions. In disciplines like Tai Chi, the Yin Yang reminds practitioners to find equilibrium between opposites within themselves and the world around them. The two dots show that there is always a bit of one element within the other, fighting styles must draw on a balance of both brute "yang" force and subtle "yin" yielding. The Yin Yang is seen on uniforms, school emblems, and texts as an icon of core philosophies underpinning martial arts.

In Japanese martial arts, the Katana sword is one of the most iconic symbols. Its elegant, curved shape and razor-sharp blade make the Katana an effective, lethal weapon demanding precision and skill. The Katana is a signature weapon of disciplines like Iaido and Kenjutsu, which teach students the specific techniques of drawing, cutting, and sheathing the Katana. More broadly, the sword represents important samurai virtues that martial arts aim to instill courage, loyalty, skill and honour. Students of Karate, Judo and other arts bow to the Katana as an object of respect. The sword is seen as a weapon to defend the weak and uphold justice when wielded by a true warrior. Even today, the Katana remains an important symbol of Japanese martial culture.

In Chinese martial arts, the tiger represents speed, power, and ferocity. Tiger style Kung Fu mimics the tiger's ripping, tearing movements with heavy claw shapes. Other animal styles like the crane, snake and monkey embody different qualities; but the tiger is respected as the mightiest beast. Practitioners aim to channel their explosive strength. Tiger symbols on uniforms or in training spaces inspire students to unleash their own inner beast. But the tiger also has deeper meaning. His strength comes not just from aggression but from subtle skills like patience, timing and balance. Training in Tiger style improves externally visible attributes like strength, and also inner qualities of discipline and wisdom to control one's power.

Though breaking boards or bricks may seem like a mere physical feat, it often carries great symbolic meaning in martial arts. The striking surface represents life's obstacles and breaking it proves one's determination to smash through barriers. While intimidating, breaks require proper technique and mental control; they teach students to channel fears into determination. High-profile breaks, like ice breaks or spear-hand breaks, have added meaning too. Ice represents the calm mind needed in the heat of battle. Spears represent penetrating obstacles by focussing one's force. The ceremonial act of attempting difficult breaks in front of classmates or masters is a rite of passage representing the student's future journey. From inner blocks to roof tiles, what gets broken reflects wider lessons on power, resilience and confidence.

Weapons training is included in many martial arts as both a practical skill and symbolic practice. Though some weapons like Bow Staffs or Sai have a functional purpose in combat, working with weapons has philosophical meaning too. Drawing circles with Nunchaku represents the continuity between movements. Repeating kata sequences with Kamas or Swords embodies the consistency and discipline needed to master techniques. Weapons expand the reach of one's limbs, acting as channels through which energy flows. Training with traditional weapons like Throwing Stars, Kusarigama and Polearms keeps antique skills and heritage alive too. Respecting weapons reflects wider codes of conduct, honouring the responsibility that comes with strength. Beyond just demonstrating skill, weapons imprint culture and values for generations to come.

Snake style movements are found across Asian martial arts like Chinese Kung Fu. Practitioners cultivate winding, fluid motions to mimic the snake's smooth attack. The snake represents qualities like speed, precision, spontaneity and constant motion. Its sinuous spine and rapid strikes inspire students to flow between techniques without hesitating. Like a snake shedding its skin, practitioners must be ready to adapt and grow. But the snake also represents inner strength through softness and relaxation, not just aggression. Snake stylists aim to exude menacing energy to intimidate opponents, neutralizing them with swift, unexpected attacks and coiling traps. Through this multi-layered symbol, the snake teaches strategic fighting and personal development simultaneously.

Though often seen as a means of organizing students by skill level, the colour of martial arts belts carries deeper meaning in many disciplines. The iconic white belt represents innocence and purity of intentions upon starting training. Progressing through colours like red, brown and finally black symbolises gaining skill, strength and mental maturity. Great grandmasters still wear pure white belts to show their eternal student mindset. Different stages inspire different virtues: white innocence, blue perseverance, purple honour, brown skill and black proficiency across all attributes. Belt systems grew organically, with colours adopted from judo by Funakoshi's Shotokan karate system. But groups like BJJ use stripes instead to downplay hierarchical obsession. Whatever the style, belt colouration keeps students striving upwards through focus, respect and discipline at each skill level.

Across every culture, symbolism plays a key role in enriching disciplines like martial arts. Whether ancient weapons denoting warrior virtues, animal styles teaching strategic skills or icons like the yin yang demonstrating deeper wisdom, these symbols guide practitioners along the journey physically, mentally and spiritually. Simple images allow beginners to access complex concepts on their path towards mastery. By diving into the layered meaning behind symbols, students keep traditions alive, understanding exactly what martial arts teach beyond just self defence in the external sense. Most of all, these icons inspire students on a profound internal journey as ethical, cultured individuals.

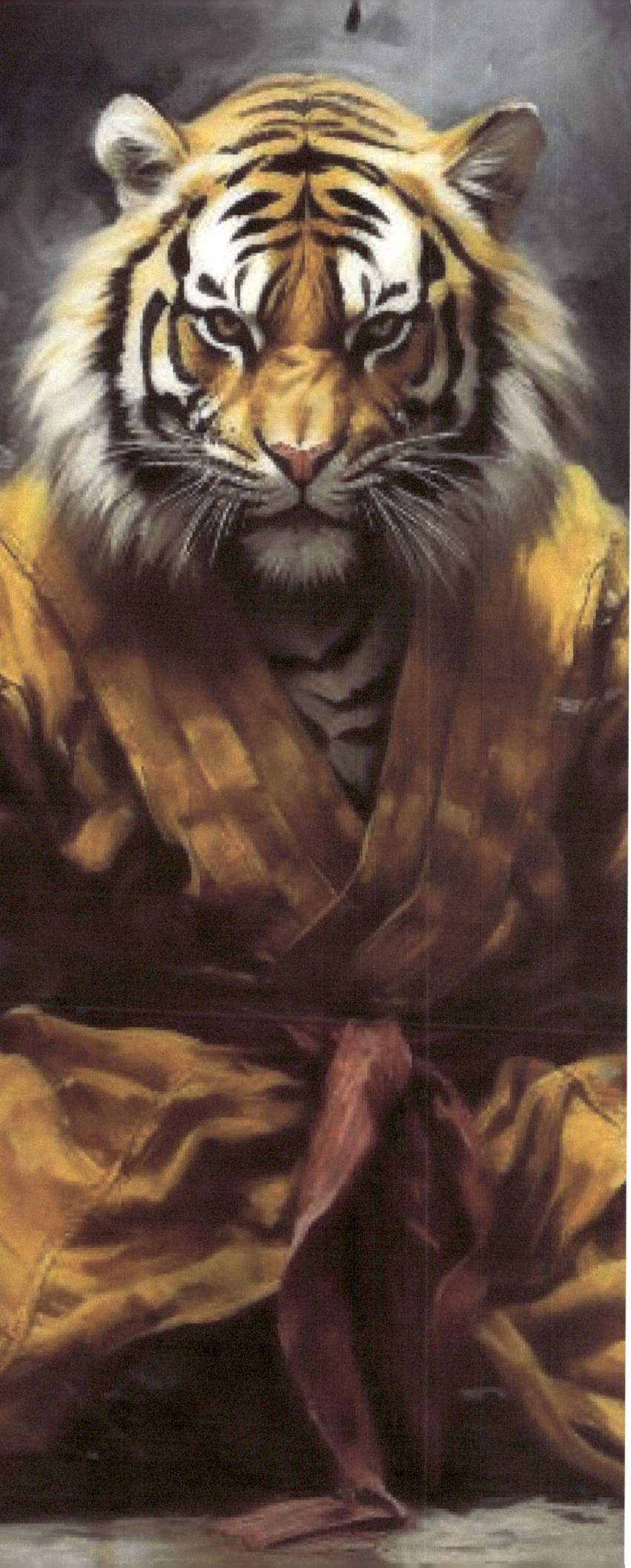

How to Survive Your First Month of Jiu Jitsu

by Sheryl Sumugat

Pat yourself on the back for taking the first step. It is the hardest. Now that you're at the foot of the mountain, it's good to know what to expect, for you'll undoubtedly encounter struggles that will make you feel like throwing in the towel.

Here are six tips to help you survive your first month of training in Jiu Jitsu.

1. Accept that you are Jon Snow.

Jiu Jitsu is Game of Thrones and you are Jon Snow—you know nothing. You are there to learn, and it's okay. No one likes to be the only noob in a room full of colourful belts. But unless you leave your ego at home, you'll only feel frustration and defeat. Stepping on the mat with a fixed mindset sets you up for failure. Instead, start with a blank slate but with a growth mindset. Jim Kwik's book "Limitless" talks about how learning difficulties can be a by-product of our ego and limiting beliefs. Like Jon Snow, you have to admit to knowing nothing so you could start learning and eventually become the hero of your own story.

2. Have a meaningful reason why you want to learn Jiu Jitsu

Make it meaningful. It doesn't have to be a tear-jerker but at least deep enough to help you get through the occasional lack of motivation.

Unless it's something meaningful to us, we tend to easily give up on a goal. Jiu Jitsu is one of those forms of disciplines that takes determination, courage, and grit. If your purpose is just to have fun and lose weight at the same time, then you're better off doing Muay Thai or Boxing. Don't get me wrong; I'm not saying they are inferior to Jiu Jitsu but they are not in the same category. Jiu Jitsu is physically invasive and even triggering to some. If you're the type of person who hates being too close to a human or twisted like a pretzel, you'll find it hard to stick around UNLESS your "why" is deep and meaningful enough to you.

3. Take it easy.

As a mum of two, I sometimes feel like it's the last thing I should be doing. I've already got enough frustrations and stress in my life, and now Jiu Jitsu? Interestingly, my husband doesn't seem to be suffering from this affliction. I realised that the difference between me and him is that he's not in a hurry. He's not putting unnecessary pressure on himself to measure up as soon as possible. Meanwhile, I wanted to keep up so badly. Not only is this unrealistic, but it also takes the joy out of learning Jiu Jitsu.

It's only natural to want to be good at something right away. We don't want to feel like we're at the bottom of the food chain.

However, our mental state affects our performance and learning abilities. It's best to approach it with a positive and relaxed mindset. Take it easy and avoid burnout. Just like weight training, you want to go slow but steady. Trust that you'll eventually get there and stop comparing yourself to your husband who's being doing Jiu Jitsu for 13 years.

4. Tap, Susan, tap!!

I was standing off the mat when I heard a cry of pain. It was Susan (not her real name) and she was trying to get out from underneath a male blue belt. She tapped on this guy but only so lightly and only once. She's only had two Jiu Jitsu lessons, so she probably had no idea how to do it the right way — which is to tap like you mean it. Tap at least twice or until your partner gets the message. Don't be shy or afraid to let your rolling partner know that you're in pain or struggling to breathe. It takes time to get used to being at the bottom. Knowing the right way to tap can save you from injuries and losing consciousness.

5. Take charge of your own learning

Jiu Jitsu classes can feel a little bit unstructured. I found it to be daunting, at first. We are used to structured lessons; one where there's a beginning and an end. It's perfectly reasonable to want someone to hold your hand and teach you the ropes from basic to advanced. Plus, I would have preferred to hear the words "There, there, don't be scared. They're all beginners just like you,"

instead of "Watch out for that blue belt. He almost put Susan to sleep." Unless you can afford a personal trainer, like Zuckerberg and Musk, gyms don't usually follow the school format. That is why it's important to take charge of your own learning. Before a session, have a goal in mind, document your progress, seek other keen white belts, and ask higher belts for advice.

6. There is no end to learning.

There's really no such thing as, "surviving your first month". It's just a lame phrase by some lame writer. You can always come back after a break. Jiu Jitsu won't break up with you like your jealous ex who left because you're always at the gym. However, if you want to understand the concepts and reap its full benefits, you need to put in time and effort. It's not a one-night stand, it's a marriage.

There are other tips out there to help you stay on the course, but I find these to be the most helpful ones in my case. It's so easy to lose motivation when you see reels on Instagram that show how good some people are. Self-doubt creeps in. "Am I ever going to be as good as them?"

My husband revealed to me one day that he's not always excited to train, that he feels inadequate too sometimes. To a beginner like me, it was enough to know that someone like him feels like a total loser too on the mat. We usually just see the result and not the process.

Finding Focus Through Wing Chun

Chip has been practicing Wing Chun, a Chinese martial art, since 1998. Now 48 years old, he credits the art with providing mental health benefits beyond self-defence and exercise. Chip suffers from hypomania, a mental health condition characterised by periods of high energy, impulsiveness, and a reduced need for sleep. He has found that Wing Chun helps provide stability and focus to counterbalance the chaos of hypomania.

"I train Wing Chun as part of my mental illness therapy," Chip says. After being hospitalised, he wrote about his journey in a published article. His instructors then encouraged him to submit a conference presentation proposal on Wing Chun, which led him to speak about rotation and simplicity at The Sydney Kung Fu Conference in 2023.

"With my mental illness, my brain is chaos, so I have to just think one thing," Chip explains. This singular focus embodies Wing Chun's first principle: simplicity. By concentrating on the basic tenets, Chip can regain awareness when hypomanic thought patterns intensify. The four other Wing Chun principles – directness, practicality, economy of movement, minimum brute force – build on this foundation.

In a video interview linked below, Chip says, "I am at a point where I have learned the forms, in terms of the sequences. Now I am just whittling away, improving how to do them. I always think, simple, rotate and go." This mantra, along with word lists, helps him execute techniques correctly and redirect chaotic thoughts.

Word lists promote concentration for martial arts and other facets of life. "I create word lists to help me with not just kung fu, but when dealing with stress and my mental illness," Chip says. "Simple tasks like packing a bag to go travelling. I use a line from them all the time."

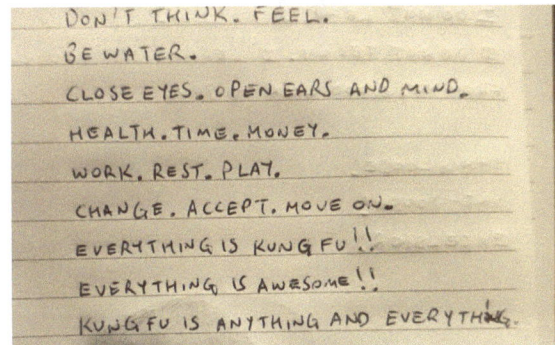

While initially struggling to align Wing Chun and mental health management, Chip now shares his story so that his practices of mind-body awareness might empower others as well. By sticking to the basic principle of simplicity, complex challenges can transform into flowing progression.

See Chip's Interview with Ryan at https://youtu.be/ezYTBVk--Bg?si=G0Et3eubhR4i1Yiy

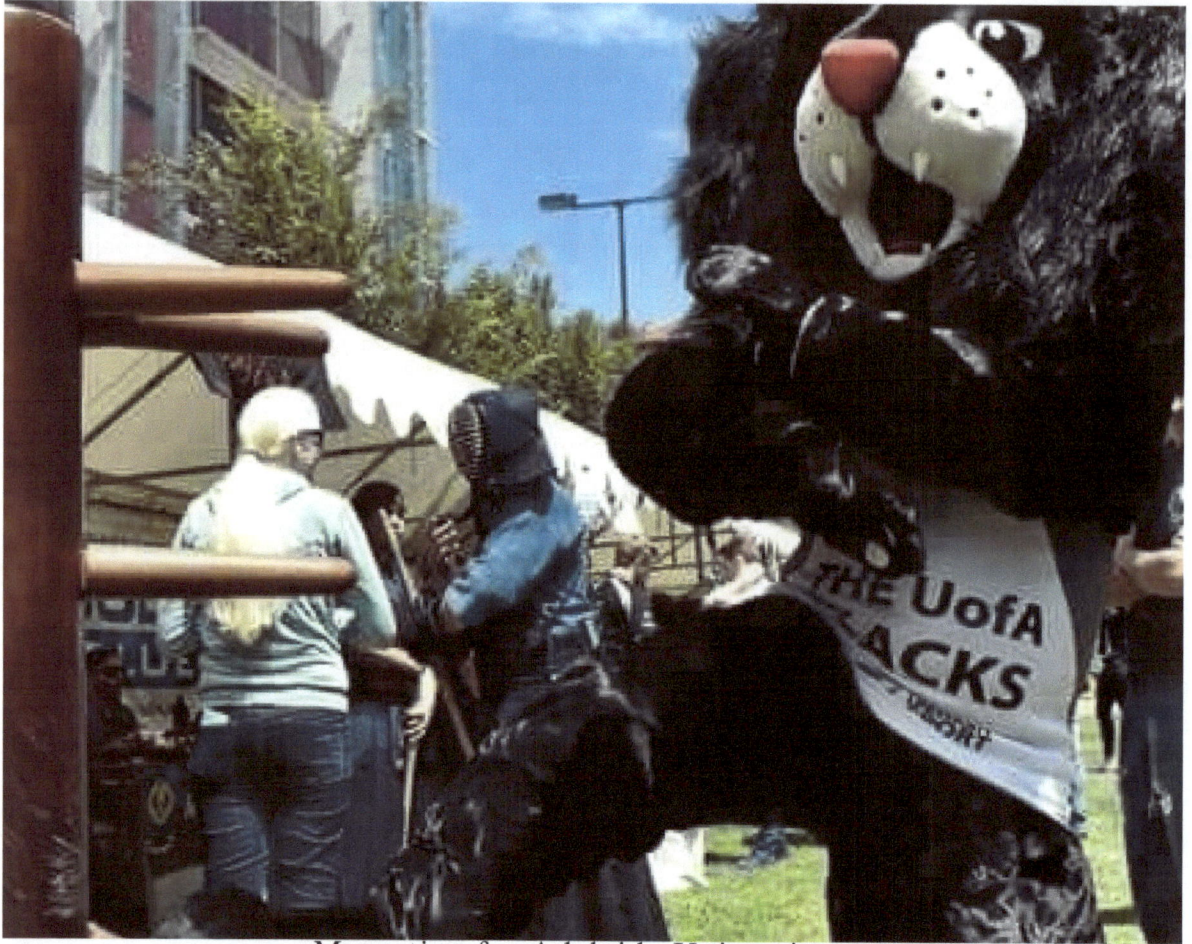

Mascoting for Adelaide University

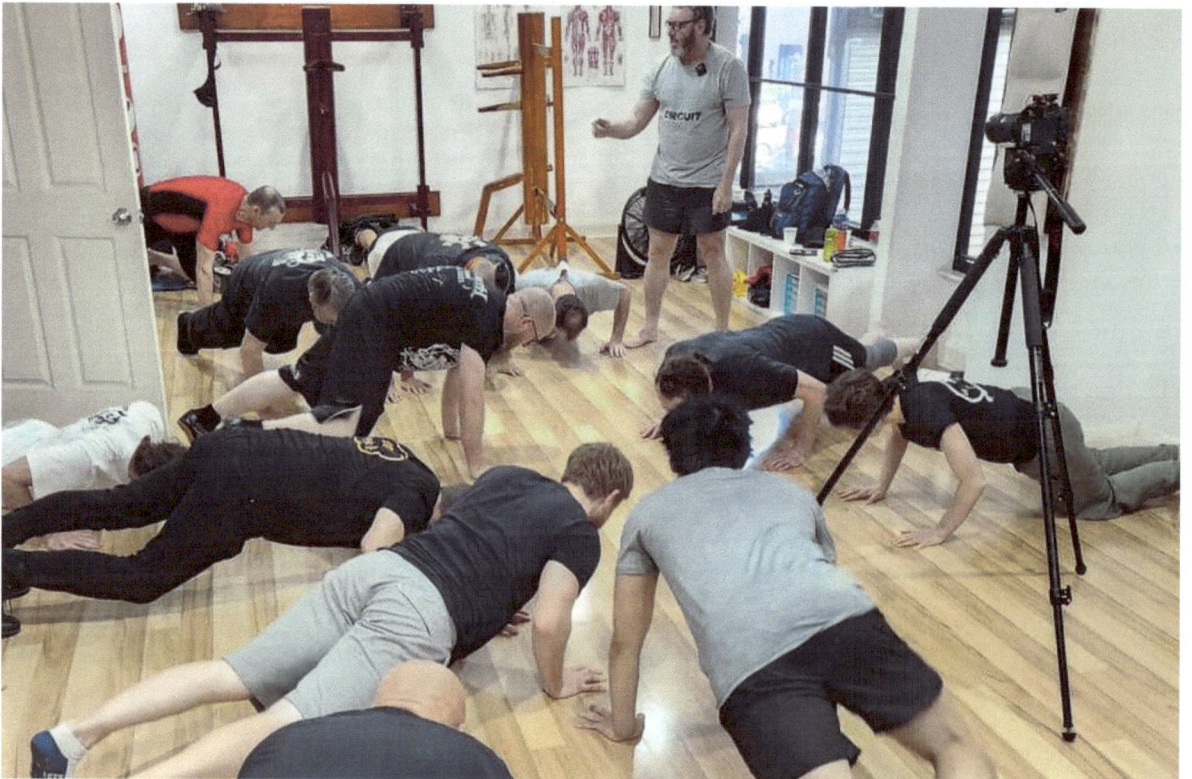

Chip Instructing at Sydney Conference.

Safeguarding Standards: Prioritising Child Protection in Martial Arts Training

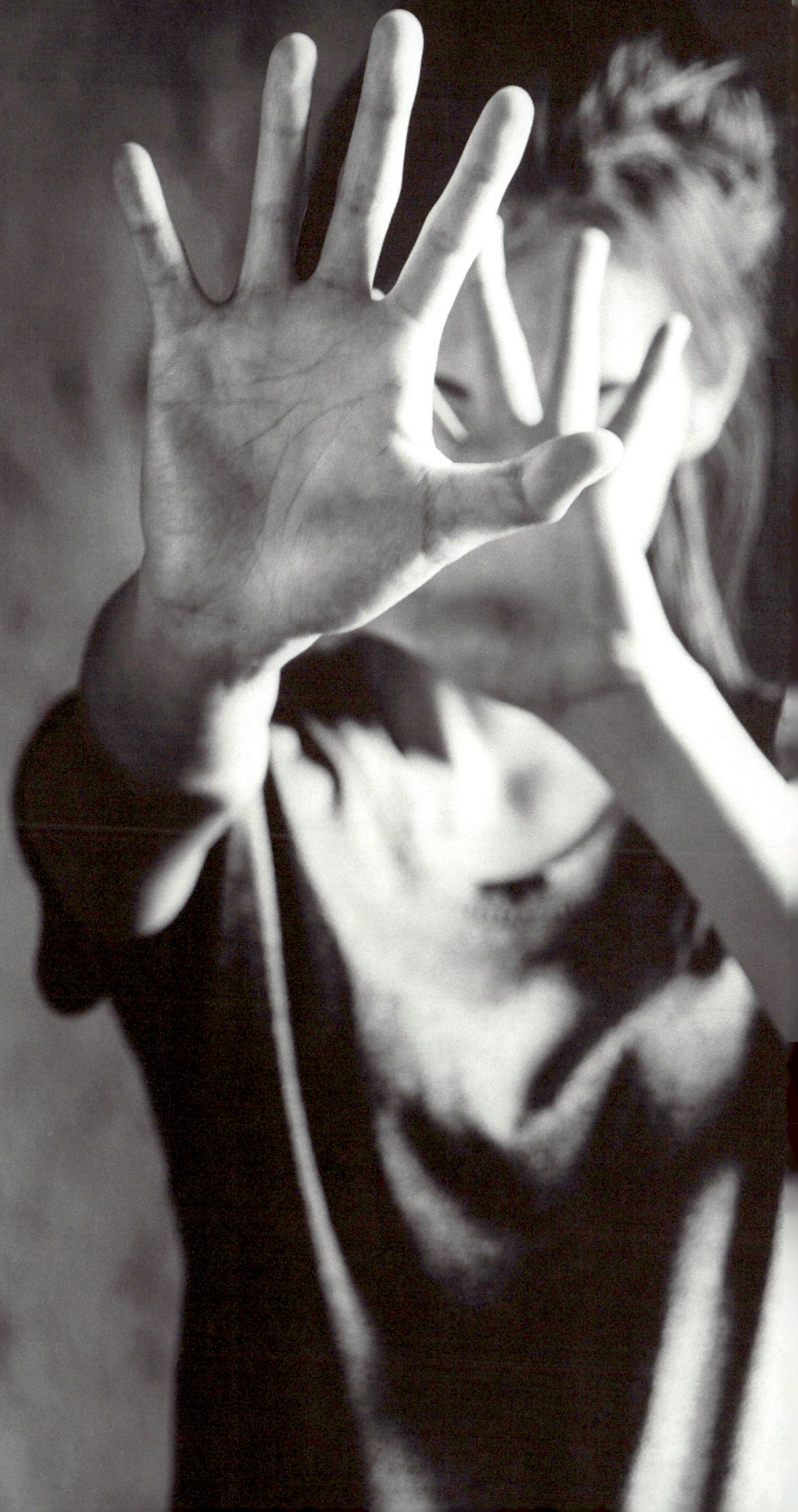

Martial arts instructors undertake an enormous duty of care by teaching children. Alongside imparting physical skills, coaches become influential role models shaping students' personal development. It is imperative every instructor upholds stringent codes of conduct and safety policies to avoid any perceptions of impropriety when working closely with youth. By internalising ethical principles, following mandated guidelines, maintaining transparency, and addressing issues head-on, martial arts mentorship can foster enriching experiences.

Instructor Responsibilities

Teaching martial arts skills empowers students to protect themselves and gain confidence. However, instructors hold disproportionate authority that can be abused without proper policies. Unfortunately, global scandals have highlighted alarming rates of sexual abuse spanning youth sports, religious groups and education settings. Martial arts are not immune: high-profile cases feature instructors that leverage their status to groom victims. Beyond overt assault, seemingly mild behaviours like inappropriate touching during corrections or suggestive jokes can constitute misconduct. Even false assumptions create damaging suspicions.

Research shows robust prevention policies dramatically reduce harm. Best practice begins with instructors introspectively recognising their duty of custodianship over children's wellbeing.

Coaches serve as guardians throughout training sessions, tournaments, or trips. Legal mandates require acting on suspicions of neglect at home. Beyond physical safety, instructors guide young people's personal growth during impressionable development. Your role demands placing students' welfare first with reverence.

Understand how power differentials, isolation and trust enable abuse in any setting. Talk openly with teaching staff about upholding conduct policies and emphasise safety culture. Encourage bystander action so everyone watches for worrying behaviours. Provide anonymous reporting channels for students and families. Recent royal commissions show systemic complicity through silence; so enable voice.

Overall, a proactive, transparent and accountable coaching approach builds trust that you take moral duties gravely. Make child protection a living conversation, not just static policies. Foster an environment where people feel safe questioning judgement calls. If anything raises concern, overcorrect through external consultation, documentation, and full transparency.

Relevant Legislative Requirements

All Australian states and territories mandate staff working with children acquire clearance verifying background checks. Exact requirements for martial arts coaches vary across jurisdictions regarding:

- Scope of roles necessitating clearance
- Specific checks conducted, from identity verification to professional misconduct charges
- Validity time frames before rechecking
- Portability of clearances when moving states
- Exemptions for volunteer parents or short-term visitors

Ensure full legal compliance specific to training context and location by consulting state commissions overseeing these schemes. Certifications must be renewed every few years. Check if additional club policies require verified clearance like reference checks. Enlist probationary measures for new hires still awaiting processing.

Beyond background checks, further laws dictate codes of conduct when dealing with children. All states criminally penalise grooming behaviours eroding boundaries to enable misconduct. Familiarise yourself with grooming typologies like targeting vulnerabilities, flattery, normalizing touch, driving wedges between child and caregivers, or institutional gaslighting; denying harm. Generally sexual activity, inappropriate contact or communication with persons under legal age constitutes criminal child abuse, especially when using a position of authority. However, even non-sexual harassment or bullying behaviours may break discrimination, child protection or OHS laws.

Overall, legislative duties require proactively identifying and mitigating any misconduct risks in training environs. Conduct exhaustive risk reviews considering potential hotspots for isolated one-on-one interactions. Assess overnight travel, change room configurations, private offices and other vulnerabilities. Embed safeguards like mandatory staff clearance, rotating attendants, parent access rights and incident management protocols. Update insurance, document policies and brief all new members to evidence due diligence. Stay appraised of legal adjustments by liaising with peak bodies and regulators.

Upholding Ethical Boundaries

Beyond mere rule compliance, championing children's wellbeing requires sound judgement and moral action from all staff. Uphold the highest codes of role model behavior. Articulate and internally reflect on where lines exist professionally, personally and ethically for appropriate conduct in context. Open dialogue builds a common understanding of boundaries organisation wide.

While positive coach bonds can greatly nurture youth, improperly close affinity risks fostering unhelpful emotional dependency. Maintain clear generational separation between adult caretaker and child.

Do not socialise privately, share overly personal information or foster inappropriate familiarity. Kids may project assumed connections from projected stories of hardship, for example; redirect them to talk to the school counsellor instead. Staff should discuss great role models or needs with parents directly and refer complex issues to youth experts, not play therapist.

Physical corrections pose another high-risk domain requiring judicious protocols. Only use strictly necessary touch for safety and communicate intentions clearly. Ask permission, give options between demonstrations or alternatives like visualization, and allow withdrawing consent at any time. Empower students to protect bodily autonomy. Coordinate guidelines for spotting, adjustments or supports across all staff, so consistency builds trust. Integrate oversight like assistants, parents watching or open doors attending 1:1 training. Stop contact immediately if any discomfort is exhibited. Make sure outdated practices face scrutiny, however entrenched, if safer modern alternatives exist.

Similarly, tightly control change room, travel and social event exposures. Prevent unsupervised mixing of child and adult domains through coordinating rosters, parent helpers, purpose-built facilities with sightlines and codes of conduct encompassing offsite contexts.

Overnight trips warrant thorough parent waivers and supervision plans. Discuss dilemmas arising around photography, gifts, alcohol or rooming pragmatically as a staff. Maintain sheer professionalism as the default.

Transparency & Issue Management

Despite best efforts, concerning suspicions or accusations sometimes arise requiring careful resolution. Move promptly to understand events fully from multiple perspectives without blame. Document fastidiously while avoiding leading an interrogation. Formal processes will apply depending on incident severity, but always reassure the upset child, then parents. If the accused staff member denies allegations, clarify the next actions: they should step down temporarily while external agencies investigate for community assurance.

However, governance should address simmering culture issues that enabled perceived failure. Revisit risk controls and staff briefings to identify gaps, refresh awareness. Reconsider past complaints through new lenses for patterns. Boost bystander training so potential issues get named early by teammates, not bottled. Strengthen feedback channels welcoming input. Review hiring practices and probation periods for new staff – look for screening improvements. Basically show that the club learns from apparent breaches.

In worst case scenarios involving prosecutions, balance member sensitivities against defamation laws. Seek expert guidance communicating with families given judicial processes limit disclosures. Maintain suspended contact with accused and continuity for remaining students. Appoint temporary senior coaches as needed if prime leadership is accused. Above all, believe children and families expressing concerns, then support experts leading a formal resolution.

In rare cases of false allegations, processes to reintegrate and heal both accused staff and the reporter still apply. Trauma healing comes first. Falsely accused coaches equally deserve the restoration of status, so reaffirm revised understandings. Enable dignity-preserving returns and continuity of training for all affected.

Protecting children's wellbeing must form the cornerstone of any martial arts program involving youth. Instructors carry profound custodial duties equipping young people with skills, ethics and personal strength. By internalizing the gravity of responsibility over care, proactively addressing risks, embedding oversight accountabilities, responding judiciously to concerns and upholding moral exemplarity across decisions, coaches can foster enriching training environs where people call out small issues early before harm occurs. Yours is an honour-bound role shaping lives – uphold this with devotion.

For more information visit:
www.playbytherules.net.au

A New Year: A New You

Setting Martial Arts Goals For 2024

by
Amy Lynch

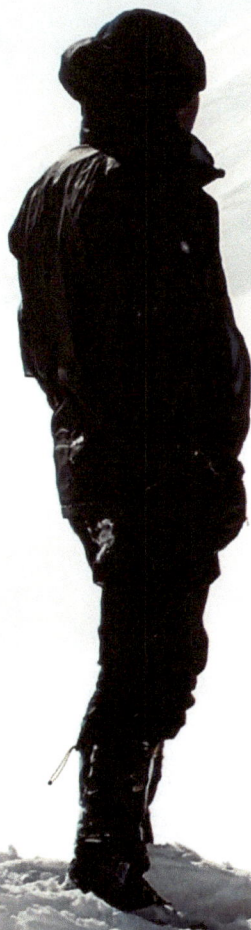

A new year brings a fresh start and opportunities to better ourselves. As martial artists, the start of 2024 is the perfect time to set meaningful goals that will improve our training, technique, mental strength, and more. Committing to thoughtful, realistic resolutions will help motivate us and enrich our journey in the martial arts.

Evaluate Your Commitment Level

Before setting specific goals, take time to honestly assess your current commitment to martial arts training. Are you giving it 100% effort every class? Do you train consistently several days per week or has your attendance dropped off? Outlining your level of dedication will help shape resolutions that target areas needing work. If you've been slacking on practice lately, resolve to attend a minimum of two to three classes every week.

Set Strength and Conditioning Goals

Improving physical conditioning should be a priority for most martial artists. The stronger and more fit you become, the better you'll perform techniques and forms. Set concrete goals around strength training, cardio endurance, flexibility and coordination. Aim to nail basics like being able to hold a solid horse stance for 60 seconds, execute 20 clean push ups, or stretch deeply into a full side split. Outline a training regimen focused on problem areas and commit to following it.

Outline Technical Skill Goals

Set resolutions around the specific techniques and skills you want to polish in your martial art this year. Planning thoughtful goals will provide a roadmap of areas for improvement. Be detailed about stances, blocks, kicks or forms you want to sharpen. Resolve to train twice a week one-on-one with an instructor to tidy basics and learn more advanced moves. By becoming a better technician, you'll feel less stressed in gradings, tests and sparring.

Improve Your Mental Game

Physical goals shouldn't override mental, emotional and spiritual goals on your resolution list. As martial artists we know that becoming mentally strong is just as critical as mastering fancy kicking combinations. Consider resolutions around building grit and focus. Develop relaxation skills like imagery, deep breathing, repeating affirmations or meditation. Read books and watch videos from great teachers on cultivating patience, calmness under stress and developing an unbeatable mindset.

Adopt a Growth Mindset

Sports psychology research shows that adopting a "growth mindset", where people believe their abilities can be developed through dedication and hard work, leads to greater achievement over those with a rigid, fixed mindset. Resolve to view your martial arts progress as a long-term accumulation of small wins through sustained effort.

Be patient with yourself by celebrating little victories rather than demanding instant expertise. Over time tiny gains compound into great improvements. Stay positive through occasional setbacks by focusing on the overall upward trajectory.

Set Inspiring Goals

Choosing resolution goals with personal meaning will fuel motivation. Setting out with the objective to finally earn your black belt for instance, provides a compelling vision. Break that major goal down into smaller milestones around technical expertise, teaching qualifications, judging certifications and time commitments to keep you steadily advancing through belt levels. Signing up to run a marathon to raise charity funds through your dojo also makes for inspiring goal-setting. Get clear on what matters most for you.

Buddy Up for Extra Support

Finding comrades to join you on your quest towards elevated martial arts skills and personal growth helps keep motivation high during the inevitable ups and downs. Initiate a year-long training partnership with a like-minded student. Check in regularly to review progress and cheerlead each other on. Partners can spot weaknesses, recommend drills, teach each other new techniques, plan healthy meals together pre-training, visualize winning nationals as a team - the shared journey will deepen camaraderie and support.

Review and Readjust

As you move through the months, remember to review resolutions quarterly rather than just setting-and-forgetting them. Life throws curveballs requiring flexibility to modify goals. Have small victories given you confidence to raise targets higher? Or are some resolutions needing to be re-evaluated if unrealistic or meaningless? Be prepared to tweak goals, ditch what isn't working and add inspiring new ones. Consistent review and adaptation is key to keeping your 2024 martial arts resolutions on-track as the year unfolds.

By taking a thoughtful approach to goal-setting this New Year's, you can expect great leaps forward in your martial arts journey during 2024. Stay committed through ups and downs, focus on incremental gains achieved from sustained effort, and partner up with like-minded students for extra motivation and accountability. Adopting this resilient, positive mindset will help you become the powerful martial artist you aspire to be. Now bow in, and let's begin!

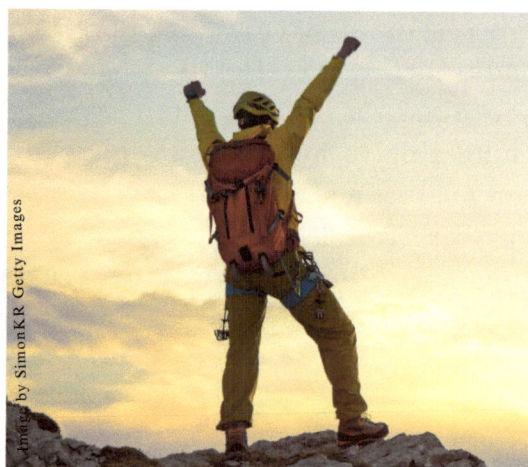

Image by SimonKR Getty Images

Strong Hips - Strong Practise
Essential Yoga Poses for Martial Artists

by Maria Francis

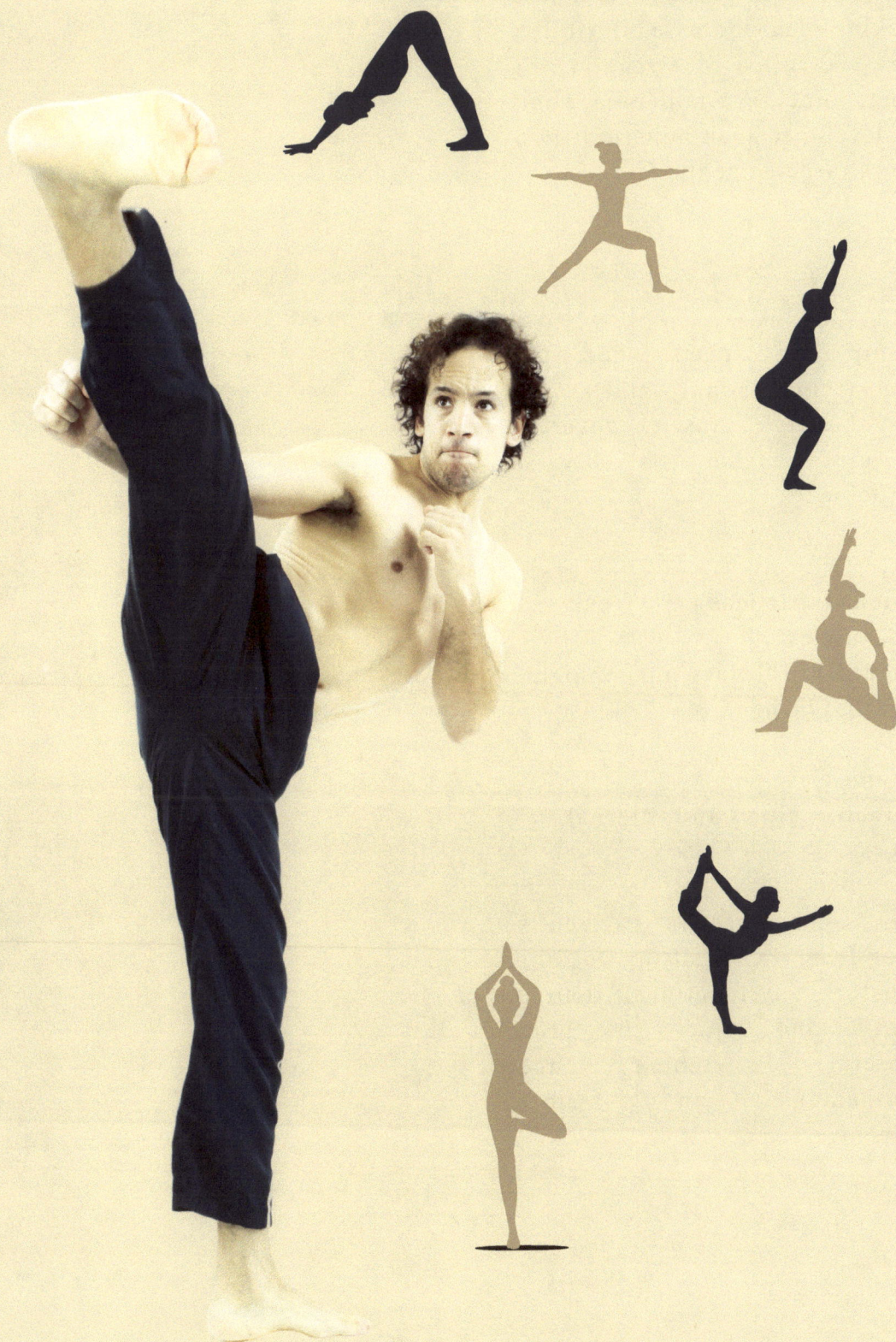

In martial arts like Karate, Tae Kwon do, Kung Fu, and mixed martial arts, powerful kicks and stable stances require mobile, sturdy hips. Tight hips limit range of motion and predispose practitioners to injury. Focused stretching can increase flexibility while targeted strengthening protects joints. For millennia, yogis have developed such holistic fitness through targeted postures.

The hip joint forms where the femur (thigh bone) meets the pelvis. Multiple muscles covering the joint enable its diverse positioning.

Common restrictions arise from:
Tight muscles:
Shortened hip flexors, inner thighs, piriformis, IT band

Weak muscles:
Underactive glutes and external rotators

These imbalances frequently develop from lots of sitting, leading to postural dysfunctions, limited mobility, and injury risk. But purposeful stretching and strengthening can restore alignment.

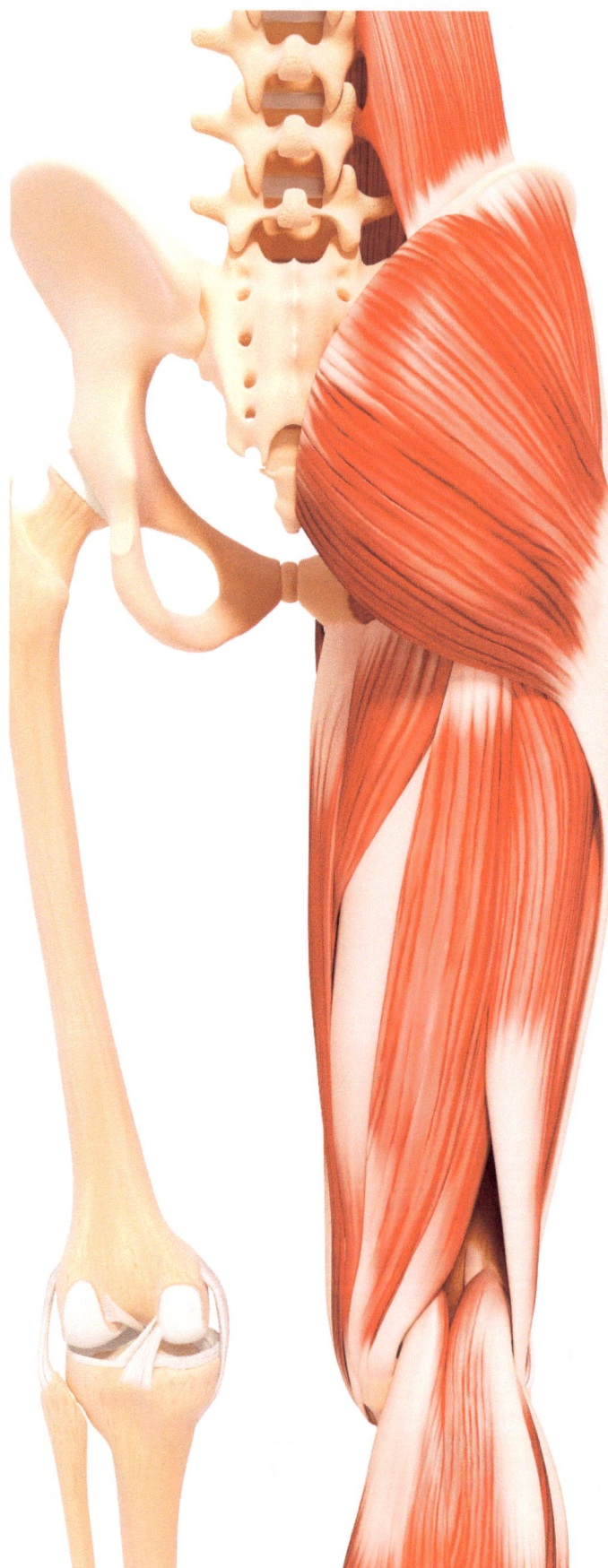

Image From Science Photo Library

Setting Up A Productive Practice

Despite variances across schools, common principles maximise progress:

1. Warm up first
Light cardio and dynamic moves lubricate joints before stretching.

2. Move slowly with control
Rushing overstretches tissues, risking damage. Ease into poses until you are feeling tension, not pain.

3. Prioritise stability
Proper alignment and an engaged core prevent compensation and injury.

4. Relax and breathe fully
Stressed and shallowed breathing exacerbate tightness.

5. Sequence thoughtfully
Alternate challenging hip openers with gentler recovery poses.

6. Listen to your body
Discomfort signals change, let pain prompt modification. Customise as needed.

Essential Poses for Hips
Incorporating these essential poses into warm ups, cool downs, and standalone practices keeps hips primed for martial arts. Move through sequences fluidly with control, advancing the depth gradually, over time.

Knee-Down Lunge
Targets: Hip flexors, quadriceps

From hands and knees, step right foot forward between hands, descending back knee to the floor with toes tucked. Ensure front knee tracks over ankle, keeping hips square. Engage core, relax shoulders down. Hold 30 seconds to 2 minutes per side. Intensify stretch by raising both hands overhead on inhale. Repeat on the other side.

Benefits martial arts by: Mobilizing tight hip flexors from sitting, deepening front stances.

Pigeon Pose
Targets: Outer hips, glutes, piriformis

From downward facing dog, slide right knee behind right wrist placing leg at 90 degree angle/your right shin is now parallel to your mat. Lower hips toward floor with back leg extended. Keep hips square, engage core. Hold 1-3 minutes per side breathing deeply. Modify by stacking shoulders over hips or placing chest on block if hips are elevated. Repeat second side.

Benefits martial arts by: Opening outer hips and loosening piriformis for higher kicks and better recovery.

Half Frog Pose
Targets: Adductors (inner thighs)

Lie on back, bend knees and place soles of feet together, letting knees drop outward. Actively press feet together while encouraging knees toward floor. Breathe fully for 1-2 minutes. For variation, raise feet onto bolster placing weight on thighs to deepen stretch.

Benefits martial arts by: Stretching closed hip angles for better side-stance mobility and kick flexibility.

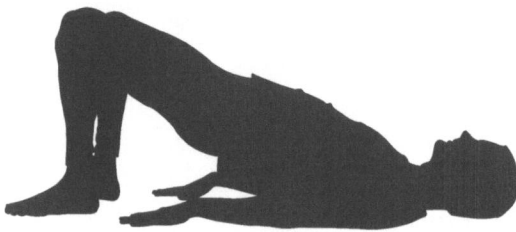

Bridge Pose
Targets: Spinal extensors, hamstrings, hips

Lie on back with bent knees and arms at sides, palms down. Exhale and lift hips up into bridge, extending through to the knees. Compress core and tuck chin, straightening back as much as possible. Hold 30 seconds to 1 minute before lowering down with control. Repeat 2-3 times.

Benefits martial arts by: Strengthening spinal erectors and glutes for balanced hip extension supporting powerful techniques.

Standing Bow Pose
Targets: External hip rotators

Stand holding support for balance. Bend right knee, grasp ankle with right hand and extend leg out to side while bowing torso slightly left. Keep raised leg in line with hip and prevent forward tipping. Hold for 30 seconds, repeat both sides for 2-3 rounds.

Benefits martial arts: Strengthens external rotators for knee control in stances and kicks.

Downward Facing Dog
Targets: Hamstrings, calves, hips

Come to hands and knees then tuck toes under, straighten legs and lift hips up and back to form an inverted V shape. Ground hands with weight in palms, straighten legs while pressing heels down. Hold 2 minutes, pedalling legs out one at a time to open hips.

Benefits martial arts by: Lengthening posterior chain, building hip and shoulder mobility for techniques requiring extension.

Seated Forward Fold
Targets: Hamstrings, lower back

Sit with legs extended. Bend knees slightly, extend spine then hinge straight at hips to fold forward, reaching for feet. Hold toes to sink chest deeper or place hands underneath thighs with arms extended. Breathe fully for 1-2 minutes gently increasing depth.

Benefits martial arts by: Improving hamstring flexibility to allow better hip motion and reduce injury risk from poor mobility.

Single Leg Deadlift
Targets: Glutes, hamstrings, balance

Stand on right foot, shift weight into heel. Soften left knee and hinge straight at hip crease, extend left leg back while sweeping right hand forward. Avoid rounding back, keep chest lifted. Hold 5 breaths each side, building repetitions for added challenge.

Benefits martial arts by: Engaging glutes in hip hinge pattern, improving stability for single leg stances and kicks.

Bridge Leg Lift
Targets: Glutes, hip stabilizers

Lie on back with knees bent, feet on floor, arms at sides. Exhale to lift hips up into bridge position, keeping chin tucked and core braced. Holding bridge, slowly straighten then lift right leg several inches keeping foot flexed. Hold for 10 seconds, lower leg with control. Repeat left side, perform 3 sets total.

Benefits martial arts by: Activating glutes in lifted leg position for core control during hip-dominant kicks.

Crescent Lunge with Twist
Targets: Hip flexors, external rotators

From downward dog, step right foot forward outside right hand rotating back foot at slight inward angle. Lower back knee down, grounding through feet. Place left hand on outside right thigh, right hand reaches up for twist. Repeat other side. Hold for 5 breaths each round.

Benefits martial arts by: Expanding range of hip rotation and external torsion required moving between techniques.

Consistently practicing these essential poses builds mobility and stability from the ground up. While challenging at first, gradual opening enables greater control through expanded ranges of motion. Be sure to tailor sequences for your current abilities and recovery needs while progressively increasing the difficulty.

Beyond yoga, integrating self-massage, foam rolling, and manual therapy addresses tissue restrictions. Remember to strengthen hips through bridge variations, clam shells, and single leg Romanian deadlifts too. With balanced flexibility and strength, martial artists can channel more power and fluidity through grounded hips for diverse techniques.

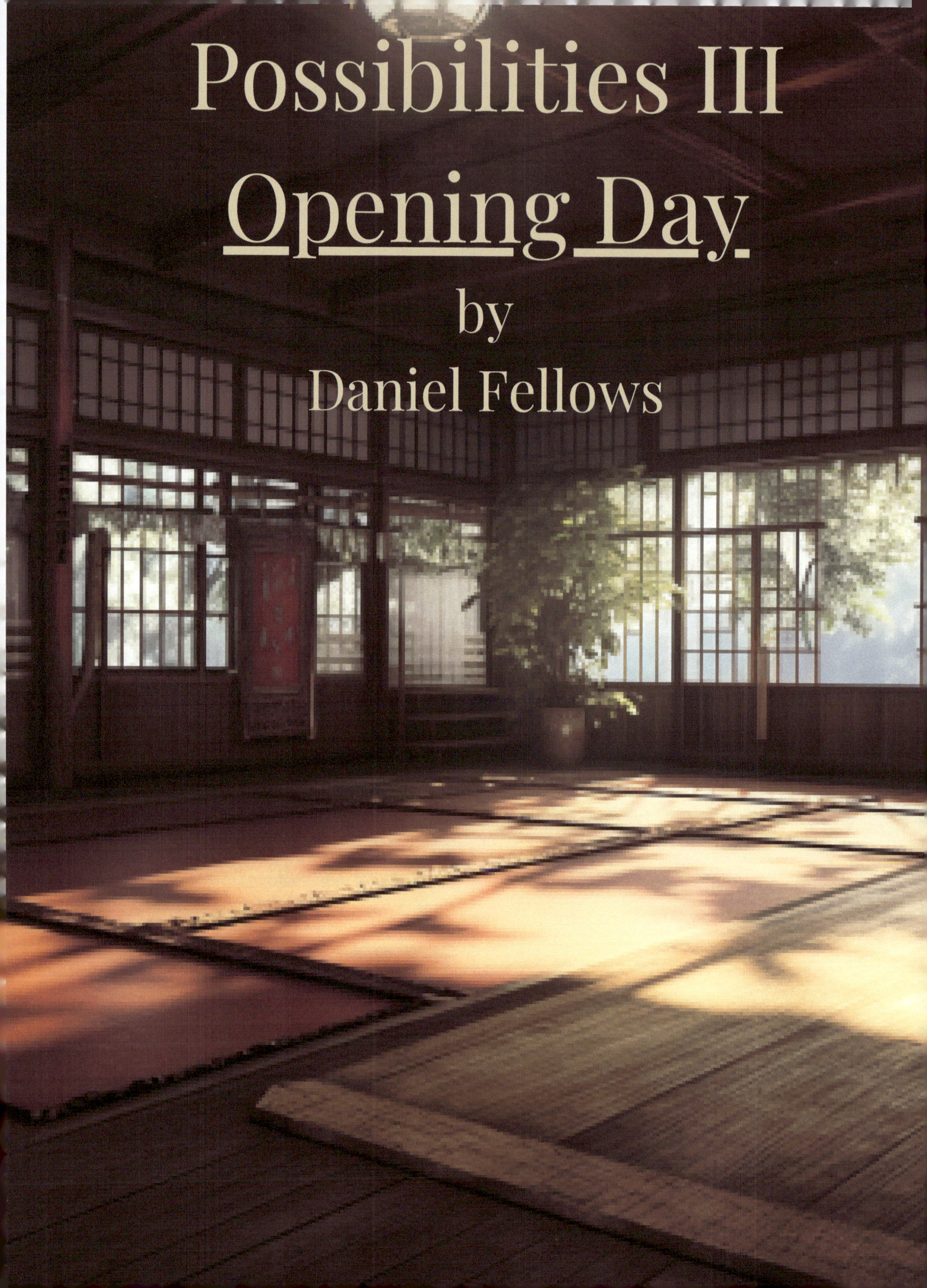
Possibilities III
Opening Day
by
Daniel Fellows

The clean-up and restoration of what Brian and Kaylee had slowly begun to call the studio was slow and arduous. Brian focused primarily on the physical destruction and wear and tear of the walls and floorboards and even water damage in the roof cavity. He spent an inordinate amount of time crawling around on his hands and knees tending to the areas that needed the most amount of attention. Gradually, the damaged and worn surfaces, both seen and unseen, of the studio were replaced and revitalised. On more than one occasion, Brian contacted the owner and was reimbursed because of the money he had spent. He figured he was doing a huge service to the owner of the building by spending the money on doing up the studio.

Kaylee, however, spent most of her attention on the studio itself. Cleaning, mopping, removing graffiti and anything else she could do to make the studio seem more presentable. The progress was slow. But worth it. The date, however, loomed.

For the longest time, Kaylee had bugged him for an actual date for their opening day. On lunch breaks, before and after their days had begun, over dinner, she would often ask her father what date he had in mind.

"We have to open soon, dad," she said rather bluntly after one particularly hard day of cleaning. "I've already ordered Gi's, belts and some sparring mitts."

He mumbled to himself and nodded noncommittally.

"The front banners are due during the week, and I've already contacted several sources about advertising and marketing. Right now, the local newspaper seems the best option available to us."

He nodded again and rubbed his chin with the back of his hand. His thick beard stubble sounded like coarse sandpaper. Kaylee felt like she was talking to a brick wall. Over the past several weeks, he had been like this; withdrawn, non-communicative. She had seen her dad like this in the past, but not for a long time. She tried to think back to when she had last seen him like this. And then it hit her. Several weeks before their move and just before he had to close the dojo. He had been depressed and withdrawn. Very similar to now.

"Is everything okay, dad? Anything on your mind?"

He didn't respond for several moments. The silence in the car was palpable. He shifted in the driver's seat, adjusted his hands on the steering wheel and glanced at Kaylee. He gave her a small, wan smile.

"Just thinking about whether this is going to be a success." He returned his eyes back to the road and swallowed heavily. "We've already used a lot of financial reserves, and I know we have to open soon to recoup some of those expenses."

"There's only one way to find out," she said, placing a hand on his shoulder.

He returned her smile and an old family favourite saying sprang to his mind. "Sink or swim, right?"

She laughed. "That's right, dad. Sink or swim. We've already had loads of interest and enquiries. And I have started a waiting list. There are mums and dads out there who have been waiting for something like this to come to town."

Brian nodded, a little livelier than before

"This is going to be a success, dad. One way or another. Even if you help one child, one family. It all helps."

"As always, you're right."

"You're only just discovering this? Now what about that Opening Day date?"

The following week went faster than she should have liked. With over two dozen things to do, she was busier than she had ever been in her life.

Making spreadsheets, finalising a working syllabus that catered specifically for young children, liaising with contractors to install the studio banners and newspapers for the advertising launch. Plus, a million other things. Later Kaylee looked back with amazement, and she wondered how she survived everything with how hectic her life was.

The day came. Their First Day. Their Opening Day. And as Kaylee promised, the phone calls and memberships followed. First one, then three, and then sooner than she had expected, the first junior's class was nearly full. Glancing down at the membership name list, Kaylee couldn't believe it.

Brian had decided their first class should start at 4:30 pm. Not too long after school finished and plenty of time for the youngest of students to have dinner, wind down and go to bed, ready for the next day.

Brian, standing by the closed door, glanced down at his watch, played with the latch of the locked door, and then looked down at his watch again. Kaylee hadn't seen her father like this since... well, for a long time. He was beyond excited. He was eager for the class to begin. Kaylee watched as he glanced down at his watch for the umpteenth time.

"Just open the door, dad. Being several minutes early won't matter will it?"

"He smiled, embarrassed, and unlocked the door. "I guess not," he said.

He barely had the door open all the way when a small face appeared around the corner of the door.

"Is it time for the first class?" asked the little boy. He walked in slowly, followed by his dad.

Brian shook his hand and they introduced themselves. More parents and children filtered into the class. Looks of eagerness and unabashed curiosity adorned their faces.

"Let's line up, shall we?"

Some of the children glanced back at their parents and they gently encouraged them to follow the instructions of the man in white pants and jacket, with a black belt.

When he had them in a semi-straight line, Brian took to the front of the class.

"Hello, class. My name is Sensei Brian. Welcome to your first karate class. Despite this belt I'm wearing, we're all equal. Just remember, I used to be exactly where you are now. I'm just a guy teaching you what I was taught by my Sensei many years ago."

There was brief chatter among the students.

"Let's begin shall we?"

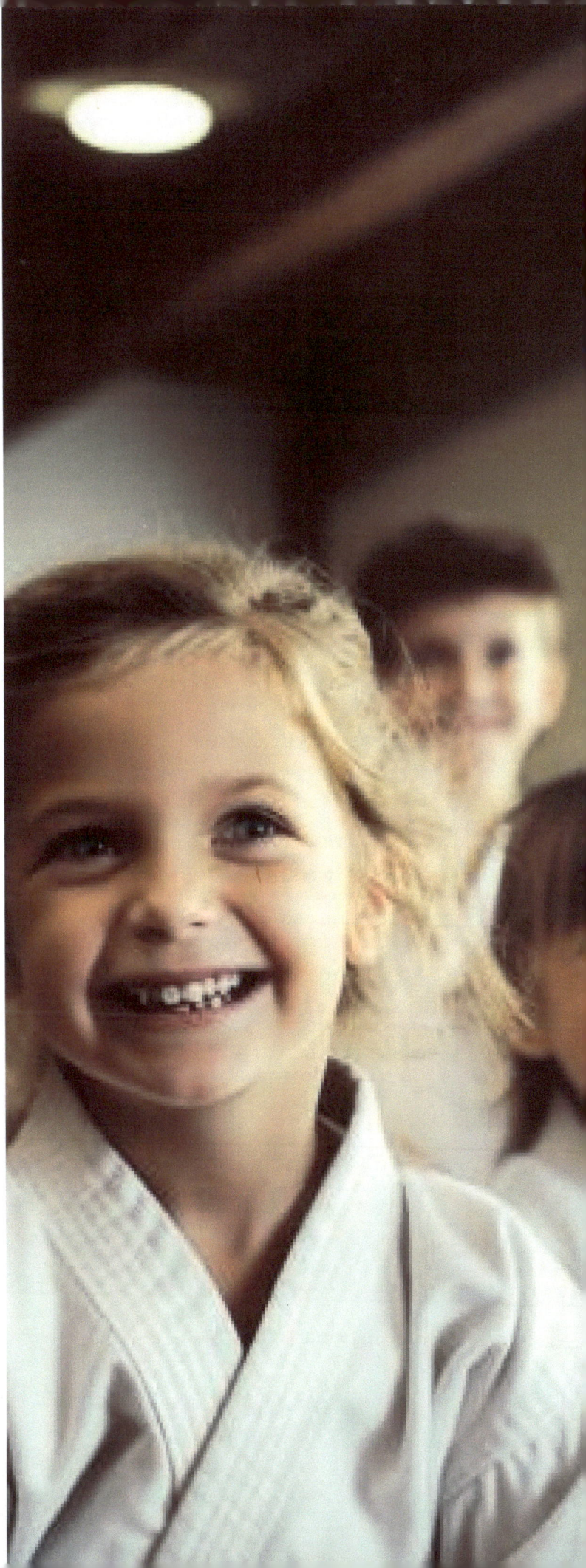

Write for Us

We want your authentic story, your journey and the reason WHY you love what you do. Below is a list of suggested topics. It is not exhaustive, so if you have an idea that we haven't come up with yet, drop us a line: training tips; technique workshops; style origins;kids in ma; training fuel; style anatomy; family pages; instructor profile; keeping it real; and more...

We are a quarterly magazine that celebrates and inspires a broad community of Martial Artists across the country. Our goal is to support all MA practitioners. Both instructors and students are encouraged to share their personal experiences, triumphs, and challenges within the style they love.

We feature interviews, rants, research, photography, projects and editorials that are respectful to all styles and are keeping in line with our magazine's inclusive philosophy.
Just as no two styles of Martial Arts are alike, our writers should have their own unique voice and tell their story from their own perspective. We encourage you to speak your truth.
Don't worry if you feel that your writing is not up to scratch, just tell us your story, your tip or your instruction the best way you can and our in-house editor will do the rest.

Email your submissions to info@martialartsmagazineaustralia.com (text in .doc) and (photos in JPEG).

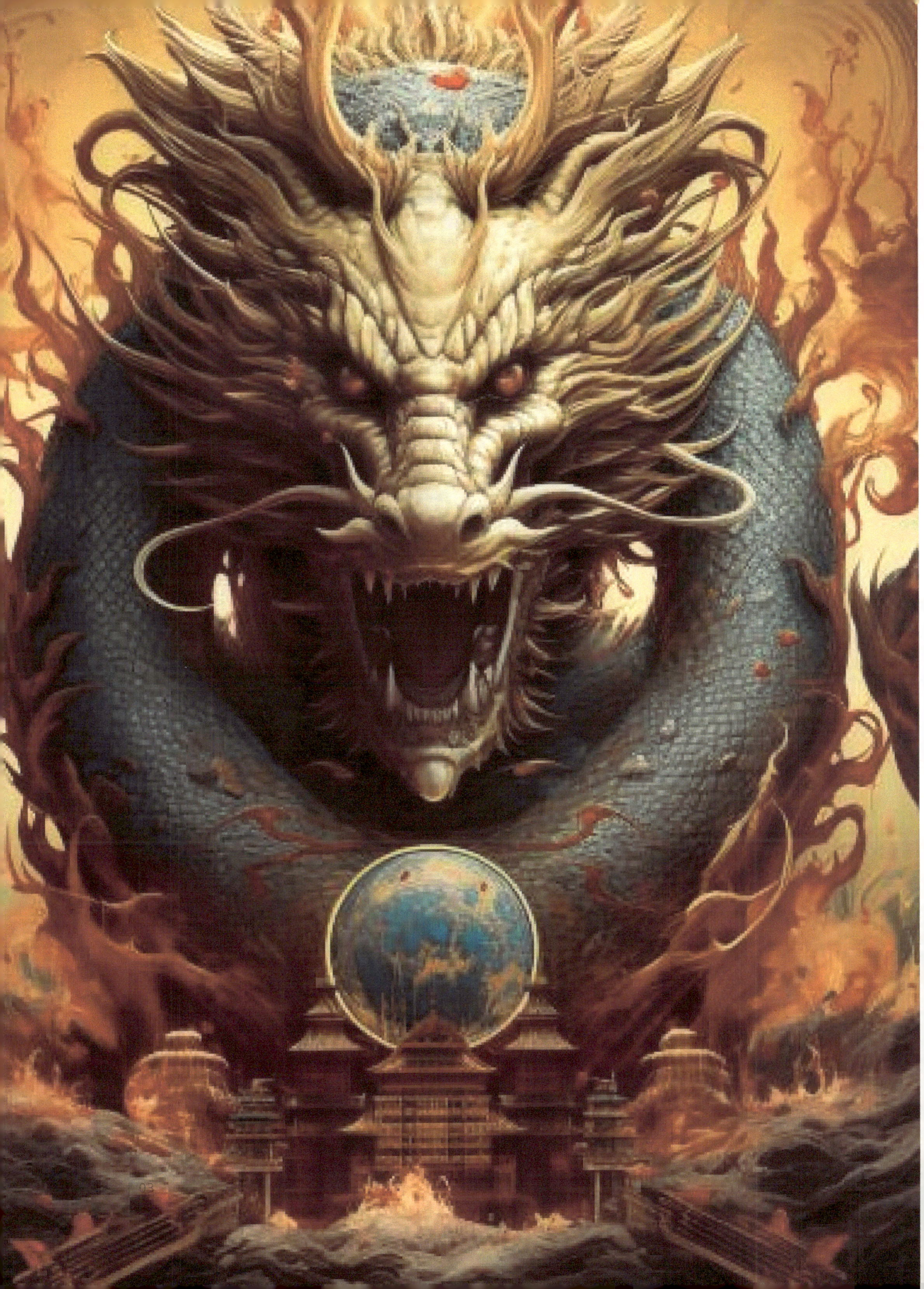

www.ingramcontent.com/pod-product-compliance
Lightning Source LLC
Chambersburg PA
CBHW061136030426

42334CB00003B/63